A Desert Daughter's Odyssey

A DESERT DAUGHTER'S ODYSSEY

For All Those Whose Lives
Have Been Touched By Cancer—
Personally, Professionally
or Through a Loved One

SHARON WANSLEE

Copyright © 2000, Thomas Charles Fensch.
c/o New Century Books,
P.O. Box 7113, The Woodlands, Texas, 77387-7113

Library of Congress Number: 00-105715
ISBN #:   Hardcover   0-930751-00-0
                 Softcover   0-930751-02-7

Cover photo by Paul Olle,
The Gallery, Huntsville, Texas

This book was printed in the United States of America.

CONTENTS

1

FORT APACHE WISDOM

"There ain't any of us gonna get outta this alive . . ."
Old Cowpuncher's Proverb

Tucson to Texas —

Nearly all the advice my wise and witty cowboy father gave me about life was true. He was wrong only once—maybe twice—that I recall, but maybe that's because times have changed so much since he grew up on my grandfather's ranch.

As early as I can remember he used to tell me, "Nothin's constant except change," and "Whatever you do, treat ever-*body* exactly like you want'a be treated goin' up the ladder o' life, 'cause you're sure gonna meet ever' *one* o' those sonovaguns comin' back down"—all delivered in his soft West Texas drawl.

Actually my grandfather's ranch lay between the forks of the Black and White Rivers in central Arizona, adjacent to the Fort Apache Indian Reservation, but all the ranchhands were from West Texas, so my dad grew up talking just like them. My grandmother 'Rene and my Aunt Florence used to get so tickled when they'd tell me about "Baby Clyde Dear" standing out by the corrals with the cowpunchers, scuffling his boots in the sand, laughing and leaning over to spit as though he had a "chaw" of Bull

9

Durham in his mouth just like the big boys. He not only picked up their soft, easy drawl, he absorbed their dry piercing wit, summing my worlds of philosophy, experience and home-spun psychology in just a few colorful, understated words.

Most of his sayings were about the business of living, but once in a while he'd throw in one about business—"If you can't make money off your friends and relatives, who in the hell *can* you make money off of?" And it was funny how anybody who did business with my dad became a friend so well did he treat them—from monsignors and millionaire cowboys to men down to their last dollar and less hope. He was even right about the business of dying when he'd say with a rueful grin— "One thing's for sure, there aint' any of us gonna get outta this alive." But my all-time favorite expression of his was one I heard all throughout my awkward growing-up years, whenever a streak of bad luck seemed to hang on longer than seemed fair—"The sun don't shine on the same dog's back ever' day," he'd tell me.

I couldn't help but smile at that one as I rocked on my back porch while I watched and listened and breathed in the Fall. Life had brought me from my native Tucson to Houston and then north to East Texas by that time, and I sought times to steal away in solitude. I loved the feel of the silky, cool air on my skin as I watched the falling, swirling leaves of oak and sweet gum and hickory. They fascinated me more than budding spring blossoms, maybe because I'm a desert woman. In the Arizona desert, autumn is gentle and filled with light and brings a blessed end to the sweltering, suffering heat of summer, but it never offered the glorious pageantry of the bountiful woods of the Big Thicket. I lost myself completely in the autumn breezes as they started the swaying of new silver plumes of pampas grass and moved on to set leaves dancing and shimmering in the sun. Stronger gusts roused their falling patterns of copper and rust and burnished brass into a symphony of rustling, soaring sounds. I loved crackling leaves underfoot as I walked. I would zigzag in crazy patterns on my path to crunch the biggest oak leaves.

Spring seems so silent. I can hear the fall; but the sound is not the knell of death or finality or "not being." It's the whispering promise of renewal, shedding the old to prepare for the new. And with the sound comes a joy, a peaceful, settling-to-the-earth kind of joy. Later, to see the craggy outlines of the bare trees is to witness their true character—stark, absolute, enduring life, with all excess stripped away—like the desert.

Amid all these sights and sounds and the purifying smell of the crisp, smoky autumnal air, I almost forgot for a moment or two the ever-present dread that destroyed my equilibrium along with my capacity to breathe; it brought such a shadow of sorrow and depression I could scarcely see.

Some say autumn naturally brings sorrow. Even Hemingway once wrote that you expected to be sad in the Fall, that part of you died each year when the leaves fell from the trees. Part of me died then—in that time of harvest, that time of rich maturity that should have reflected the fulfillment of all that had gone before—for that's when the stalking nightmare finally confronted me. Nineteen years earlier, my beautiful, gentle mother, Sara, died—lingeringly—of cancer. At the age of 35, I was struck by the same reaper's blade, in the same place—over the heart. The terror of that specter gripped me, immobilized me.

Even though I like to think of myself as a writer, words would not come. Before, words flowed freely, easily, spontaneously, whether writing for small town newspapers or spilling impressions of life's paradox into journals—I'd been keeping them for seventeen years. But that October day I put away my pen. I couldn't write. I couldn't even talk.

All my life, images and humor jumped so glibly from my tongue an Irish friend of mine named Joe once advised in his purring brogue, "Sure an' don't ever be kissin' the Blarney Stone, Sharon—the world isn't ready yet." But that day my mouth was struck as mute as my typewriter. I couldn't even sleep, at least with any peace at all. And although much of my life had been spent bumping into door jambs and dipping my sleeve in guacamole, I foundered, fumbled and stumbled more than ever.

It was a classic replay of the Ford/Rockefeller story. First Lady Betty Ford wouldn't have detected her own cancer, had not Vice President Rockefeller's wife, "Happy," suffered two mastectomies. And because my friend had a biopsy, I first discovered I had cancer. I was writing feature articles for the *Huntsville Item* and city editor Rana Shields wrote a series of articles about the dread disease. During her research she discovered a lump in her breast and immediately scheduled a biopsy in one of the big Houston hospitals. While awaiting her confrontation with the surgeon, Rana's words were positive and calm, her work as creative, thorough and under-the-wire as always. Only her pencil turning and twisting the cowlick at the crown of her head into auburn tangles betrayed her anxiety. I silently marveled at her seeming composure, as I watched the burnt-red bird's nest steadily grow, and I wondered if I could have stayed so outwardly serene.

Her biopsy came—benignly—and left scarcely a conscious afterthought in my mind. Yet, deep down, I knew I was long overdue to check my own body. For years, when confronted with conversations, articles or programs about cancer of any kind, especially breast cancer, the beginning of my mother's nightmare, I quickly changed the subject, turned the page or snapped off the television. I didn't even read Rana's series. If I didn't think about it, hear about it or read about it, "It" simply could not happen to me.

I handled death and dying with the same insistent denial. Logic alone should have told me that no matter how much tuning out and turning off I managed, "It" not only could, but most decidedly *would* happen to me. How many times had I heard my Fort Apache cowboy father dryly observe, "There ain't any of us gonna get outta this alive . . ."

Neither could I run from cancer by closing my eyes and ears. I had to do an abrupt about-face and march straight into the hells of cancer and dying, trying to conquer my fear of each.

Paradoxically, I had to face death first.

Survival Rule #1:

Now is the time to become more open, more receptive, more inquiring into the ways of hope and survival than you have ever before been in your life—you are entering a new and different world.

II

FUNERAL: THE END?

I felt a Funeral, in my Brain,
And Mourners to and fro
Kept treading—treading—till it seemed
That sense was breaking through . . .

Emily Dickinson (280)

"You've got to be kidding!" I told him. Please be kidding, I prayed. I don't think he's kidding.

Michael Leggett, managing editor for the *Huntsville Item* had just assigned me the odious task of researching and writing an article on the costs of funerals. Michael usually was kidding, but this time he seemed oblivious to my rampant necrophobia. He calmly folded his hands across his ample stomach, tugged on his mustache and said, "I'm dead serious. Would I joke about dying?"

Day after day I researched. For a week and a half, I gritted my teeth and traipsed in and out of morgues and funeral homes—those for the black folk and the mansion-like one on the hill for the white folk with its cavernous display room filled with caskets in muted mauves, empire blues, royal reds and every fabric, style and price imaginable. These long, colorful boxes ranged from a modest felt-covered pine model for $450 to the heavy ornate, cast-copper sarcophagus for $20,000.

Each day Michael asked, "Where's the funeral story?"

I overlooked nothing in undertaking, from the training necessary for morticians to the cost of flowers for funeral and cemetery.

"Where's that story?"

I investigated costs of various types of headstones and crypts. I even delved into the costs of cremation and the required urns for the resultant ashes and the optional "columbariums" to hold the urns. I must have filled 15 to 20 legal-sized pages with lugubrious notes.

And through it all, Michael kept asking, "Where's that funeral series?—it's gotta be a series by now."

But I couldn't write the article. After learning everything Michael wanted to know about funerals, I was more afraid than ever. Since beginning the research, I'd been unable to sleep. When I did manage to doze, nightmares awakened me. The most frequent and frightening?—I would be putting to use an empire blue casket long before I'd written my great all-American novel and lived my great all-American life.

The next time Michael asked, I confessed. At his suggestion, I sought out Dr. Richard Cording, who taught a seminar called "Attitudes on Death and Dying," at Sam Houston State University.

Hearty and stocky with steel-gray, close-cropped curly hair, Professor Cording looked much like an ex-football player, but wasn't. His gaze was direct and his words straight-arrow. My nervousness gave way before his sympathetic kindness, sensitivity and warmth, which made me wonder at the time why he chose for our conversation an empty, echoing, windowless, icy-gray cubicle with nothing in it but a bare oaken table and three or four heavy wooden chairs. I explained my dilemma.

"Struggle," he told me. "Struggle with your feelings, because there's no taking death away." I had no idea how intense the struggle would soon become.

He then gave me a "death-anxiety test" consisting of 15 questions. My answer to the first question surprised me. The question read—"I am very much afraid to die: true or false?" I answered an unequivocal "False!" And through the remaining questions I discovered that all my anxieties and sleepless nights were due to the fear of "prolonged and painful illness" leading to death, not death itself.

On an anxiety test scale of one to fifteen, I scored eight, which was one-half point higher in anxiety than the average score for women, and two points higher than the average score for men—or, as even Dr. Cording pointed out, two points higher than the *professed* score for men.

"Not bad," Dr. Cording smiled at my obvious relief. He loaned me two books from his class—*On Death and Dying*, by Elizabeth Kubler-Ross, and a novel by James Agee, *A Death in the Family*. So comforting were his words, I hugged him before I skipped down the stairs from his office. So consoled as to be euphoric, I was eager to tackle those voluminous notes, to turn them into something of Life.

From that point on, the four articles became fun for me. "Funeral: the end?"—Michael titled the series, with the sub-head: "Not to the bills, it isn't." On the premise of planning my own funeral I based my lead on a recent article concerning a ninety-nine-year-old Colorado man, who had arranged and actively participated in his own "funeral" celebration, his twenty-first in twenty-five years. It seems his "last rites" using the same copper coffin but different eulogies, created the biggest bash his small town ever experienced. He claimed he wanted to hear all those good things people were going to say about him while he was still alive. And besides, he allowed, if it was going to cost so darn much, he might as well enjoy the party. Somehow that made sense to me, and the story later amused my dad.

Throughout the articles I arranged for everything from an empire blue casket covered in yellow roses, four or five extra limousines to accommodate all my family and friends from Arizona, to insurance to cover the costs. In reality I prefer a simple pine box. My favorite roses are the Arizona-sunset-flame-colored variety, but how could I admit this to Texans. The final article in the series dealt with the fears I'd unearthed in my research, and the resultant conversation and test with Dr. Cording.

Michael and Rana liked the series with its tongue-in-cheek slant and entered it in that year's state competition. I liked the articles, too, and as I'm sure many aspiring writers do, I enjoyed rereading them. But overshadowing each critique loomed the realization that I was afraid, not of death, but of "prolonged and painful illness."

For a time after my mother's death, I forced myself to go through a breast self-examination, or BSE, every three or four months, or as often as I could muster the nerve. Within only a couple of years I abandoned it completely. But one late summer Sunday as I sat reading at my desk in the bedroom and looking out through the sliding glass doors to all the healthy, thriving oak and pine trees in the sunshine, I determined to prove myself healthy. Rana had told me the easiest way to initially check your breasts was in the tub or shower because the skin is wet and slippery and fingers can slide and probe with more sensitivity. So I started running the shower.

Alone in the house, I moved in silent slow-motion as I undressed, my heart's cadence heavy and hard. I entered the shower—barely breathing. My God, my breath was so shallow and slow. Twice I shampooed my hair, and twice I conditioned it. Then I scrubbed and scrubbed from head to toe. I rinsed slowly. Then I rinsed again and stalled and stalled and stalled. I stood under the steaming water for seemingly interminable moments and contemplated my fingertips shriveling and turning into the color and texture of dried peaches, while I seriously considered the wisdom of postponing this until some other time.

"For Christ's sake!" I rasped to myself in disgust. "Will you get on with it?!" I reached for the soap and slowly circled the lathering bubbles round and round my breasts. My arm seemed suspended in space as I watched my hand put the soap back into the dish. I forced my fingers to follow the patterns of the soapy suds, tentatively, anxiously sliding and probing. "I've got to do this now!" I growled through gritted teeth. "See? there's nothing, absolutely nothing. Everything's fine. All's clear and healthy except . . . except . . . ah, God, please no . . ." I whimpered. "Please no, not now, dear sweet merciful Christ . . ." I took my hand away and leaned against the cool tiles, watching the soapy water swirl down the drain . . . trying to think of nothing but the white, sudsy, marble-like designs. Maybe if I search again, I won't find anything. I tried again. No, there's no mistaking it. Yes, there really is a small, hard— dear God, it's such a hard lump in the outside upper curve of my left breast. And it hurts, and I want to scream, but the sound dies somewhere in my chest where I can't catch my breath.

I was alone, the house empty and still. Even my two dogs, Chica and Sam, and my two cats, Miguel and Feliz, were gone, off chasing some creature or each other in the woods. I remember, because I had never felt more alone, more abandoned, and I wanted to hug their warm peacefulness and tell them how scared I was.

Instead I reached my doctor who lived only fifteen minutes away in the tiny town of Riverside. I asked if I could come by for a few minutes, sounding, I thought, calm and composed considering my panic-stricken condition.

John Halberdier was a friend as well as my personal physician. Young, in his early thirties, tall, lanky and easy-going in appearance, he was an intensely caring doctor, treating the whole person, the mental/psychological health as well as the physical. Like many doctors in Texas, he wore cowboy boots and jeans and listened to Willie Nelson. I could hear Willie singing "Blue Eyes Cryin' in the Rain" as I walked through the doorway of the small, faded white frame house John shared with a lawyer friend, who was also divorced.

Over red wine for me and black coffee for him, we talked about every subject I could think of: "Willie, country music in general, Huntsville, problems of the Texas prison system where his lawyer friend worked—everything except what I came to talk about.

John just let me talk, listening, waiting.

Two glasses of wine braver, I told him.

He reassured me, "Most all these nodules are benign." The lump in my throat began to dissolve a little. Then he told me everything I needed to know—statistics I wanted to hear and those I didn't, chances I might have and measures to take if I didn't. He even described, at my insistent urging, surgical procedures involved in both a benign biopsy and a radical mastectomy. But with the hearing, I closed my eyes, shook my head and asked if he would mind not using that word—"mastectomy." It scared the hell out of me—or into me.

In my fear I couldn't look at him while he described all those operating techniques. I focused instead on a small teakwood sculpture on the coffee table. What I at first thought to be the Japanese god of joy gradually revealed itself to be a naked, pot-bellied, grinning troll, seemingly enormously proud of his rotundity. Suddenly it seemed ludicrous, even bizarre, to talk of body parts—my body parts—with any degree of gravity with this grotesque caricature of gluttony facing me.

"Good Lord!" I couldn't help but laugh. "I thought I had problems . . ."

"Aw, that's my roommate's," John explained, red-faced, then we both got tickled. God, it felt good to laugh!

Hearty red wine could not brace me the following day for the second higher hurdle in that race of terror, the examination in John's office and an X-ray at the small local hospital. I bumped awkwardly along through those experiences as though I were performing in a surrealistic puppet show—forced through motions beyond my control, wooden with fear, a smile filed on my face, yet somehow believing through it all that this was just a bad script.

This couldn't possibly be happening in Real Life . . . at least not now. I was just beginning to find a semblance of peace. There were times I thought I'd never learn the meaning of the word, much less live it. Enmeshed in an on-again, off-again marriage that was not only unhappy but chaotic, I had almost established the groundwork to finally make a break, build my own quiet life with my son, Morris Patrick. How could these tests bring a death sentence to all that longed-for tranquillity and gentle joy?

I prayed to be spared that cup. And I was.

"Just a benign little lump that will go away all by itself," John's nurse assured me when she called the newspaper office with the test results.

Ah, God, thank You! Relief for a while. I breathed deeply. Life resumed. I didn't have to drink from the cup—yet.

Another month went by—writing, meeting deadlines for the paper and preparing for the sad, personal deadline. My pathetic plight of marriage was being resolved by dividing all the furniture, paintings and memorabilia yet one more time. Everything was set for the final separation.

In the meantime, the "benign little lump" not only did not go away, it grew bigger and more tender, frightening me beyond all telling. "Don't believe anyone," I told family and friends, "no matter their credentials, when they tell you any lump or nodule that hurts isn't cancer because "pain is only evident in the last stages of the disease." From the first moment I detected that lump in my breast, it hurt to touch it. It hurt, burned, even when I didn't touch it, and the tenderness transcended my psychosomatic fear.

I was sent first to Houston, to John's brother, Dr. Stayton

Halberdier, a family practitioner.

"I'm sure this is nothing to worry about," this older, more citified version of John tried to reassure me. "Usually a woman doesn't need to worry 'til she's about thirty-five."

"Tomorrow's my birthday," I told him, my one last thread of hope fraying badly. "I'll be thirty-five."

More soberly this time he said, "Well, often all these lumps need is just to have fluid drained from them." I tensed my toes and tried to concentrate only on them as he inserted that long, long needle into my breast—and when he began to pull on the syringe to draw out the hoped-for fluid, he drew nothing but brain-searing pain and a primal wail.

From that instant, I knew I was born into the world of cancer.

Survival Rule #2:

In the beginning you will experience shock and denial. A feeling of numbness will set in. This is okay. It's normal. Slow down and savor small moments as you go, and remember words from a wise, old cowpuncher—"Take 'er slow."

III

"Renascence"

"And all at once things seemed so small
My breath came short and scarce at all."

"Renascence"
Edna St. Vincent Millay

"My breath came short and scarce at all . . ." kept echoing through my head that afternoon when Dr. Halberdier city-version sent me for a mammogram to "Suite Z." "My breath came short, and scarce at all . . . and all at once things seemed so small . . ." The lines seemed so familiar, but for a few moments I couldn't place them. The words kept repeating over and over and suddenly I remembered the what and the why of them. The words resurged from nineteen years past, from Edna St. Vincent Millay's, "Renascence," two hundred fourteen lines all about death and rebirth, long one of my favorite poems, I'd discovered it, ironically, at the age of sixteen, the year my mother died. "My breath came short, and scarce at all . . . My breath came short and scarce . . ."

Take several deep breaths, I told myself, long and slow and sure. Use all the techniques you know: relax the muscles in your jaw and those in the neck and the shoulders and the back and the hands and legs and even the toes . . . The panic subsides. For a moment. Maybe relaxation exercises don't work if you think you've got cancer . . .

I tried again and again to think of health and wholeness

and happiness. But how difficult it was while experiencing the impersonal xerograph machine and the cold and empty room with its "condierioner" and "processor" and the cold and empty and fat technician with short, greasy, streaked blonde hair and a sullen mouth and expressionless eyes that made me wonder about her own health and happiness. I finally dismissed all thoughts of wholeness and well-being while feeling her unfeeling, dry-icy hands position my breasts for the xero-mammogram as though they were so much quivering calves liver being compressed into a package and weighed indifferently for purchase.

I remember the two copies of *People* magazine in the room. The top one, of course, featured a photo of Happy Rockefeller—and I, who for so many years had assiduously avoided any article dealing with cancer, breast surgery or dying, turned dutifully to the article about her and her two breast surgeries, as hundreds of other women in that room must have done, fearfully. A quietly smiling, wise face with eyes that reflected resignation and the inevitable knowledge of pain looked back at me from the pages. I took another deep, deep breath. I wondered how she felt to be designated the sacrificial ewe, her slaughtered breasts martyred and publicized to warn and save other women pain and death. It was because of her that Rana started her series and because of Rana that I was now sitting half-naked in this cold computer-like room reading about "Happy"—my God, *"Happy?!"*—and waiting—and scarcely breathing.

The technician came in again and without even the merest suggestion of a glance at me said, "You can go."

My God, at the time kindness and understanding are most needed, indifference bordering on hatefulness is offered. I hurriedly left her and her frigid environment, walking past the women waiting in the outer office. I saw their expressions of fear and felt sorrow for us all.

I walked out into the bright sunshine and the clear, crisp

October air that I love, and I wanted with my whole heart never to have to go back—ever again. It was good I was alone. I needed time to think, to catch my breath, to adjust to this new and disorienting world. I drove as slowly as possible to a nearby coffee shop, and over carrot cake and comforting milk, I mixed thoughts of life and death, of pain and sorrow, of joy and hope—mostly hope—until tomorrow . . .

Hope fled when tomorrow came. For I knew when I looked into the surgeon's eyes after his examination that not only had the time come to drink from the bitter cup, I was to drink to the dregs. Dr. Jose Iglesias quietly ordered his nurse to schedule bone and liver scans and bloodwork in three days and to schedule surgery shortly thereafter. When he looked back at me his eyes were moist. The doctor, originally from Colombia, South America, considered to be a "surgeon's surgeon" in Houston, told me more with his kind brown eyes than he did with his words. Although everything he said was comforting and consoling, his expression told me the situation was grave. I loved him and trusted him from the first moment not only for his gentleness and compassion, but because he could not hide from me his sorrow or his fear.

He told me what procedures he would follow: first, a biopsy, and then, if necessary, either a modified radical or a radical mastectomy—each involving complete removal of the breast and lymph nodes in the axilla, or armpit.

He explained more, but I'd heard all I could absorb. That word again—mastectomy. The syllables themselves sounded butchering to me. The air seemed suddenly close and much too warm and my breath came shorter and scarcer still.

What he didn't tell me, I'm glad I didn't guess. He had also discovered smaller lumps in the left axilla, the right axilla and the right breast indicating possible extensive metastases. And with my mother's history haunting me, how wise not to tell me. What would have been the point? I was already convinced I'd been flung headlong into an absurd dance of death rapidly gaining whirling, dizzying speed, like the Yaqui ceremonial dances I'd witnessed as a child at Easter in Tucson. Scary then. Scarier now.

I left his office, stunned. I remember stumbling down that long, long corridor in search of the exit. I walked right past it and started down another long hall before I snapped to long enough to retrace my steps. I sat in my car for the longest time, taking deep, deep breaths and trying to get a handle on all the emotions surging through me, until finally I was able to arrange a mask in place, frozen cheerfully on my face, just like those same Yaqui dancers.

Only with my priest and friend, Salvatore, did I put away that mask and let the fear and the grief break through. Only with him was I able to handle the hurt of it all as the anguish overflowed. For a very long time, not even my son was allowed to see my cheerful mask drop. I arranged it carefully back into place as I started the car, and then once again I drove as slowly and as safely as my condition would allow to a friend's office. Didn't my dad always say when you're feeling down to seek out the friends who can cheer you? They don't even need to know you are down.

Going through all the motions of saying hello to old friends and exchanging stories made me smile. Meeting a new secretary whose low-cut blouse revealed a stunning, non-stop cleavage made me nauseated. I suddenly realized what cleavage I had would soon be gone. I had to sit down.

That experience marked the moment I began to label each happening, each event in my life, "The Last Time Ever"— "The Last Time Ever in this Office," "The Last Time Ever at the Texas Renaissance Festival," "The Last Time Ever Return to the Tucson Desert . . ." The next "Last Time Ever" experience was later that night—the first time ever I attended a Neil Diamond concert.

Unfortunately, by the time my friends were able to get tickets, the only remaining seats in the Houston Summit were behind the stage. It didn't matter—such is the energy and infectious joy of Diamond's "bullfrog" voice. When I walked into that concert, still terrified from the afternoon news, I felt I was just biding time waiting for the lid to be nailed onto my empire-blue coffin. But as the lights dimmed and the multi-colored strobelights flashed and criss-crossed through the Summit's smoky blackness and the soaring strains of the old favorites began—"Solitary Man," "Kentucky Woman," and "Craclin' Rosie"—I was caught up in the sheer joy of it. Just as though I were a child again, my heart beat fast and it seemed as though my eyes and ears had veils torn from them. I could see colors more vividly, stabbingly, and hear sounds more piercingly than ever before. With "Soolaimon" and "Brother Love's Traveling Salvation Show," I wept for the "Last-Time-Everness" of it all.

Then the final segment of the show began, featuring the music from the soundtrack of "Jonathan Livingston Seagull." Dressed all in shimmering white, Diamond seemed to me a shining prophet of promise as he sang his words of overcoming. The melodies, the lyrics were all brand new to me, but I felt as if I'd always known them: "Transcend—Purify—Glorious." I thought, Oh, God, do You suppose I could?—Do You suppose I might just beat this thing? Maybe I could transcend and purify . . . and dear sweet, merciful God, wouldn't that be glorious?

Six hours after I l earned I had to have cancer surgery, Diamond's music struck a responsive chord in me. I'm grateful he came out on tour that year, ending a four-year self-imposed exile. I needed his music. I later heard Diamond say in a radio interview that his goal in each concert is "to make everybody forget everything else around them and just go crazy." He didn't make me forget. But he brought hope to the cancer-craziness, the despairing cancer-madness already growing inside me.

As soon as the music stores opened the next morning, I bought my own copy of "Jonathan Livingston Seagull." I didn't want that responsive chord to fade—ever—and I played it each time my spirits began to sag, which was often.

Back home, I told Morris what that concert meant to me. And as if sparking the will to fight were not enough, I told him how Diamond spurred me to write this book. Asking him not to laugh, I explained that every time I heard the words,

"Be—as a page that aches for a word

that speaks on a theme that is timeless" and

"Sing—as a song in search of a voice . . ."

I took them personally. The words tugged at me, pulled at something from inside me.

I wanted to speak out, to say something. I needed to write my own song that would defeat the despair and despondency and death-laden terror that is cancer—for my mother, from me, for anyone who needed to hear.

He didn't laugh.

Survival Rule #3:

Listen to your own inner body knowledge. If I had waited to have my first mammogram until I was fifty, as the American Medical Association now recommends, I would *never* have had one. *I would already have been dead for fifteen years.*

IV

Racing Time In Slow-Motion

". . . swift there passed me by
On noiseless wing a bewildered butterfly,
Seeking with memories grown dim o'er night . . ."
"The Tuft of Flowers"
Robert Frost

For the next three days, slow-motion moments hung heavily in time, and incongruously, hours raced by headlong into my past. I tried to seize those moments and hang on with teeth-gritting intensity to make them stay. My jaws were sore from the tension. But Time refused to stay in the Now. It hurtled by me in an on-going kaleidoscope of tumbling, colliding, happy-sad moments: celebrating my 35th "Last Time Ever Birthday," breaking the medical news to my father and brother in Arizona, trying to reassure them, being confronted by caring phone calls from friends and by time spent with my son.

How the tender devotion of my fifteen-year-old Morris Patrick moved me. To tell him of the coming ordeal, I called him into my bedroom. I sat in my rocking chair; he sat on the corner of the bed. I told him of test results, surgical procedures and percentages of recovery as positively, optimistically as I could manage. But I had barely begun when he fell to his knees in front of me and buried his face in my lap.

"Oh, Mama!" he cried. Not since he was a little boy— "Mama."

I held him for a long, long time, thinking how fulfilling it felt, praying I would have many more years to do so. I tried to push aside the sudden, painful realization that I was also fifteen when I learned of my mother's cancer, and that by the time I was sixteen she was gone.

"It's all right, it'll be all right," I kept crooning to him as I held him and rocked. He'd flung his glasses aside and his green-blue eyes kept filling with tears and more tears. I stroked them from his face and smoothed back his hair and tried my best not to give in to tears myself.

Morris cried for three hours more. We'd always been close—good friends as well as mother and son—but during those hours of shared fear and sorrow, we grew closer still. When the tears finally stopped, it seemed as though all Morris's strengths—spiritual, emotional and physical—rallied. His eyes were red, his face puffy and swollen, but his inner self seemed stronger, more determined. He became a primary source of energy and renewal, and he didn't let me see tears again for a long, long time.

From that point on, he spent many extra hours with me. He played games with me and tricks on me and how he made me laugh! He became serious only when he played music for me.

"Listen to this, Mom—I mean *really* listen," he'd admonish as he put yet another album on our stereo—Gary Wright's "Dream Weaver" or Peter Frampton's "O Baby, I Love Your Way." He even taped "Jonathan" so I could take it with me to the hospital. That's when I cried.

Music, lots of music, everything from Gregorian chant and Bach to Texas' Dan Fogelberg, and all of Neil Diamond, helped soothe my soon-to-be-savaged breast. Morris and I listened together.

Sharing music and sorrow and hope was the only comfort

left. The three days were gone. It was Time. All the distractions and diversions had helped me maintain a cheerful facade, but I was still the Yaqui dancer, outwardly displaying cool courage, inwardly not feeling it. Inwardly not feeling.

Numbly, and almost dumbly, I stumbled through the tests—blood, urine, X-rays, EKG—all through that first afternoon. I only vaguely remember. More tests the next day—bone scans, liver scan. More waiting. But now I fretted while stretched on tenterhooks beneath four or five flimsy white, waffle-weave blankets to combat the chill of a 104-degree fever.

What an anticlimax! A simple but virulent, kidney infection, at first latent, now raging, would delay surgery. For how long?

"It will take," Dr. Iglesias explained, "at least two full weeks to clear it up. Meanwhile I want you to go home and rest and take all of these tablets. I know they look horse-size, but that's really very dirty-looking urine."

"Oh, God . . . *two more weeks*—Probably just enough time for the bad stuff to spread completely enough that any chance I might have had will be destroyed. Two weeks of gearing up to calm down—just enough time to cure my kidneys and lose my mind. Deer Sweet, Merciful Christ—what am I possibly going to do for two more weeks?

With my next aching shiver, I decided I was too sick to care. I guessed that aching, tossing, turning and moaning a bit ought to be good for at least a few days of it. It was. And by the time I felt somewhat better, a close friend of Morris named Bill appeared at our front door—a big poster board under one arm and the biggest box of Grumbacher pastel chalk I'd ever seen under the other—like some young Navajo shaman with curing colors.

He wasn't equipped for a sandpainting, but he and Morris had a plan. In the box were four dozen shades of pastels ranging from deep ultramarine blue to the merest hint of lemon yellow. On the 3' by 4' poster board, he had sketched, with information from Morris, some of my favorite things: an enormous butterfly, exactingly drawn in minute detail, a varied assortment of flowers, three mushrooms for Irish good luck appearing whimsically in the upper corner and a wide rainbow descending behind it—all waiting for me to fill it with color, to bring it to Life.

I stumbled through words, trying to thank him.

"It's no big deal. Look at the drawing again—I wrote a poem at the bottom."

I looked more closely this time, and penciled in at the bottom of this surprising drawing was a barely discernible poem of two stanzas:

"Butterflies and flowers," I read aloud,
"and happy things,
Such is the beauty
Your thoughts must bring—

"For each in its way
Is yours to keep,
If only you now
Continue to seek . . ."

I didn't yet realize, of course, the impact that gift would have on my life, how I would "continue to seek" again and again because of this simple design. Morris and I filled it with the last strokes of brilliant color barely in time to take it with me to the hospital.

The Navajo Shaman's creation was ready to fulfill its - purpose.

Survival Rule #4:

A medical diagnosis of cancer can make you crazy. It's important to know that *this madness is normal.* There are many ways to deal with the craziness so that you can deal with the cancer—and win.

V

"A New Year"

"My Lord God, I have no idea where I am going. I do not see the road ahead of me. I cannot know for certain where it will end. Nor do I really know myself . . ."

Thoughts in Solitude

Thomas Merton

What a way to begin the New Year!—enroute to Montreal via Air Canada. It was January 1, 1977, and I'd never felt so alone. Somewhere between Houston and New York City I unfastened my seat belt and tried to stop thinking by putting on earphones and listening to music. But music only started the memories again—too many memories, so much had happened in the last two months.

Through it all friends and family and mostly Morris were always there—every morning and evening and sometimes throughout the day. During the first two surgeries, as I was wheeled away and as I came to. When I awoke the second time, I saw Morris' face—at first dimly, fleetingly. Then as I began to focus, I became profoundly aware that his face meant strength and life and hope for the future to me. I could see the "Butterfly Painting" over his shoulder. Suddenly I remembered why he was beside me.

I tried to touch my chest. Leaden bandages were all I could feel. How surprising, I thought, to feel no pain. Having probably the lowest pain threshold ever recorded in the history of womankind, it's what I'd feared the most.

The day was a haze of faces: Morris and Salvatore and Drs. Iglesias and Halberdier, the anesthesiologist and numerous nurses, who I saw periodically when I discovered that, yes, there is pain. Each time I grabbed the railing and slowly rolled over to bare my hip for another mind- and body-numbing shot, I wondered what my female forebearers would think of my frailty, especially my paternal great-grandmother whose courage was legendary in our family.

The previous night, Morris and my two doctors and two of my friends appeared in my room, one by one, seemingly coincidentally, until Dr. Iglesias began to talk. I'm glad I could see the strength and seeming serenity of my son's face when Iglesias said that the frozen section of the lymph nodes removed in the biopsy that morning revealed a malignancy. It had spread. I tried not to think, "How far?" The modified radical mastectomy would be necessary—the next morning.

"It's okay," I said. "I already knew," which was partly true. I had to go through it one step at a time. I couldn't bear being put under anesthesia without knowing beforehand what would be done—if I would awaken with both breasts or one. I had to have time to gather courage, to prepare my mind, my body, my soul.

With the reality of pain I discovered that courage was no longer needed. There is a continuum of events that sometimes carries one along despite any willingness or unwillingness to cooperate. In this continuum, I didn't have time to fully experience fear because in a hospital there's hardly any free time at all. It's always "Time for Something:" eating, shot-giving, bathing, bed-changing, bandage- or pulse-checking, blood-testing, temperature-taking, visitor- and gift- and flower-receiving, and sandwiched in-between, catnapping, if at all possible, because in a hospital there isn't much silence for sleeping.

Visitors and flowers—especially roses—cheered me considerably. On the window ledge sat two dozen long-stemmed American Beauty roses, from my father, and the single pure white rose from Morris's friend, Bill. Whenever I looked at them, I felt that peace and beauty still existed in the world despite the dark red blood draining from the hole in my chest beneath the snow-white bandages.

Those were such seesaw days—a contrast between horror and flowers, blood-red dressings and fresh green plants, between feeling vibrant and energetic, and fainting and falling flat on the bathroom floor the first time I tried to sit in a chair to bathe myself.

"You lost an awful lot of blood during surgery," Dr. Iglesias explained to me as I opened my eyes, wondering how I got from the icy-cold tile floor back into my warm bed. "We can't give you any blood to replace it because the lymph nodes are gone. We can't risk infection."

He was still talking when an orderly carried a tree into my room. My brother Patrick had sent me a seven-foot fig tree, full and burgeoning with Life. How glorious. I looked at the beauty of the tree and the gentleness and caring of Iglesias' face instead of the dressings or my blood-draining chest each time he checked the healing progress of the seven-inch lateral incision across my now prominent-rib cage.

On the fifth day after surgery, Iglesias and my favorite nurse, Dorothy, marched determinedly into the room and briskly pulled the privacy curtain around my bed. The minute I saw their faces, my inner alarm antennae zoomed to full attention and waited—vibrating.

"Why so serious?" I asked, trying to sound calm.

"Sharon, we're going to remove that drainage tube," Dr. Iglesias explained. Quietly he added, "and it's going to hurt you very much." He and the nurse looked at each other.

Once again I was so moved by his compassion, his tenderness, I couldn't take my eyes from his face. He began to remove the dressings, then he stopped. He took a deep breath and looked intently into my eyes for a moment before he began pulling the drain tube from deep within my chest.

"I'm sorry I have to hurt you." His words were almost a whisper.

He told me later that most women cry out and weep with the pain of it. I don't know a logical explanation, how such things happen. I only know that this person, who has the lowest fathomable threshold of pain, felt no pain whatsoever. I was conscious only of the tube moving as he gently pulled it and of the loving kindness in his face.

"But I didn't feel anything at all," I told him.

I remember he looked down and smiled slightly. When he looked up, there were tears in his eyes. So much for the myth of the cold-hearted, clinical surgeon.

*   *   *

I recuperated quickly. It's a family trait. My cowboy-father says it's because my Grandpa Tom was "so tough he could break broncos with a busted appendix." And he did—once— although he lay nearly dying in a hospital for the better part of a year following.

And I was cheerful. Such a good patient. I didn't look sick, and I certainly didn't act sick. I told everyone I'd had a few bad moments because of the surgery, but never a bad day. The amazing part is that I believed it myself.

No wonder Fr. Tom Monahan took one look at me and exclaimed, "Sharon, it looks as though you haven't had a sick day in your life—you look just great." Fr. Tom, a Catholic priest of the Redemptorist order, had become a good friend through marriage counseling, or maybe I should say "separation counseling" considering the outcome.

"Who did your painting?" he asked as he leaned over to

read the poem at the bottom.

I told him all about the surprise gift. "you know, as I painted it with pastels, I felt just like a second grader with a brand new big box of Crayolas."

"I didn't know you liked to work with color," was all he said, but he gazed at the drawing for a few moments longer.

After we'd talked of life in general, and health, mine in particular, he asked me what I was going to do since I probably couldn't continue working for newspapers, at least for a while. I didn't know what to tell him. I hadn't really thought about it, except I knew I wanted to work more closely with people in an environment that might give more lasting satisfaction than newspapers. Before leaving, he took my hand and prayed for me, for courage, for complete recovery. Despite his caring and thoughtfulness, I silently wondered what earthly good his words could do. What I needed was rest not spiritual rhetoric.

Too early the next morning he was back. "Sharon, this is just a thought, but how would you like to teach a course in creativity?" Before I could answer he continued, "I thought about this all night—we've been looking for someone to go to Montreal and study with a doctor who developed the course and then return to Houston to teach it. I think you just might be the one."

I was the one all right. That's why I was soaring 30,000 feet above the Earth this New Year's Day, listening for the third time to "Nadia's Theme" on the airline program. That melody always made me feel nostalgic, melancholy, lonely. My thoughts filled with the devotion of loved ones and how they stood by me all during radiotherapy—taking turns driving me back and forth from home ninety miles south to Houston every weekday—waiting and watching on the video screen from the next room as the big green cobalt machine, that I named "og," performed his powerful magic on my chest, and all during that next surgery in December, nine days before Christmas, as I was wheeled into the now terrifying operating room for another biopsy, this time in the right axilla.

Morris's smiling eyes told me the good news as I awakened. Even before he spoke, I knew it was benign. Benign! We laughed and cried—and then I vomited. That surgery made me dreadfully sick. Occurring so close to the other two, they had to change anesthetics, and I didn't tolerate the new medication at all. My terror of the cancer spreading intensified the problem, and complicating everything was my dread of the hateful anesthesiologist. Aloof, detached and very "professional"—or so he thought—he never even looked at me, nor changed expressions or tone of voice, nor would he shake my proffered hand the night before surgery. [In retrospect, I'm not sure he even blinked. Tall and wiry and totally expressionless, he reminded me of a slithery desert lizard staring down from a saguaro perch. Actually, a desert lizard has a great deal more personality and will look straight at you . . . Just to think about his cold, discomforting disdain made me feel nausea all over again . . .

"Oh, God!" I took a deep breath and pulled the earphones away. Maybe the worst is over. Here I am in an Air Canada 727, winging my way to a new world in a New Year, preparing for my first dinner of '77. I wondered what Morris was having for dinner . . .

How he and Fr. Tom pushed and pulled me to come to Montreal to study this new and exotic painting course that I was supposed to eventually teach. I tried to hedge. I didn't want to go. I tried to procrastinate. Fr. Tom dialed Montreal and handed me the phone. I tried to tell Wolfgang Luthe—Wolfgang!—that I'd have to wait until after radiotherapy to study with him. He told me I didn't. There would be two women from Berkeley starting the course the first week in January and I "should be with them." I could, he added, "learn much from them."

When I called my cowboy-father for sympathy and support, he asked just one question, "Will this help you get well a hundred percent?" I thought there was a very slight possibility, thinking of a diversion, new tactics, new interests, new career possibilities.

"Then, by God, bow your neck to the wind and get on with it." So much for a loving father's molly-coddling.

I masterminded an elaborate, last-ditch effort just to let time run out . . . At Fr. Tom's urging, Morris called to make the airline reservations, and he even reserved a little Gremlin for me at the airport car-rental agency.

"How fitting," I muttered, "a Gremlin."

There'd been nothing to do but go. Even Dr. Collins, my radio-therapist at Houston's Rosewood Hospital, assured me there would be no problem in splitting the course of cobalt treatments while I spent time in Montreal.

Dr. Vincent Patrick Collins, how I absolutely adored him, almost to the blasphemous level. My first impression of this Canadian Scotsman from Toronto was that of Albert Schweitzer with a Santa Claus smile. His fringe of snow-white hair and his bushy gray-white walrus mustache suggested he should be wearing a Scottish tam and knickers and puffing on a drooping, meerschaum pipe.

Each time he grasped my hands and pulled them toward his chest as he asked me questions, I felt as though he'd pulled me into his life with the most loving, gentle care. His hands were warm and so were his sparkling blue eyes as he peered closely at me. He inspired such confidence that each time I saw him or heard his rich, lulling voice, he filled my spirit with hope and peace.

To mark my chest for cobalt treatments, he strategically placed three pencil-point-sized dots on my uneven torso. Only three tiny dots, not the heavy black, ugly lines mapped across the body that the "Reach for Recovery" lady described, and which I've seen slashed across scalps and faces and necks of other patients, unwillingly revealing their war-zone demar-cations for all the world to see. Obviously, their radio-therapists weren't blessed with the sensitivity of a Vincent Patrick Collins . . .

. . . "Ladies and gentlemen: The captain has turned on the 'Fasten Seat Belt' sign as we'll be experiencing some slight turbulence . . ."

I fastened my belt and thought about my "Reach for Recovery" representative . . . That lovely woman from the American Cancer Society's volunteer outreach program did all and said all she could to reassure me, to help me. She even warned me not to buy any new lingerie until treatments were finished, because of her own "war-zone" experiences. Her demarcation lines had ruined all her luxurious, new silky wardrobe. This mastectomy veteran had driven all the way from Bryan, about 75 miles away, just to try to make me feel better.

We talked and laughed over hot desert chaparral tea. I smiled and told her I was grateful she came. She smiled back and told me I was the most cheerful cancer patient she'd ever met. I smiled and waved as she drove away. Then I closed the front door, picked up all the pamphlets for ordering and paraphernalia for exercising and carefully placed them in the miniature Reach for Recovery shopping bag. Trying desperately to dam the tears, I marched into the bedroom and flung the bag and its contents under the bed so *no one* could see them—*especially me.*

I started pacing. Dammit! I don't want to be reduced to a booklet—a pamphlet for a prosthesis. Jesus!—this whole experience has *lacerated my soul* as much as my body, and they hand me a cute little pulley and a chart for rope tricks and mail-order catalogues in clever packaging and that's supposed to make it *all right?* I clenched my teeth and growled and forced myself to choke back the surprising tears.

When I told Morris about it, his eyes became so sad. I couldn't bear to see him look so sorrowful, especially knowing that I caused it. I tried to cheer him with an anecdote I remembered, a story his grandfather, my cowboy-father, told me years ago that he'd read about Socrates: When condemned to death by drinking hemlock, Socrates accepted his doom, as everyone knows, stoically and with great grace. But his wife, cantankerous, nagging, old Xanthippe, bemoaned his fate, wailing, "But why you, Soc? You've been so good to Athens and all its people! You don't *deserve* to die." To which Socrates simply replied, "Would it make you feel any better, Xan, if I *did* deserve it?"

The story made him smile a little, and it made me think a lot. No, I never felt I deserved cancer. And yes, it would have made me feel exceedingly worse if I had . . .

". . . Ladies and gentlemen:" . . . Many miles and many thoughts later, the stewardess' voice brought me back to the reality of now . . . "The captain has once again turned on the 'Fasten Seat Belt' sign for our approach into Montreal . . ."

I looked out to a new crystal-white world sparkling in the sunshine below me. This must be what Siberia looks like, I thought . . . and feels like, once I had disembarked. That glittering, glacial world felt more isolated and more bitter than any I'd ever known.

Aside from the biting wind and snow as far as I could see in every direction, my strongest impression upon arrival in Montreal that New Year's Day was one of overwhelming fatigue and sorrow. I stayed at the airport hotel for a day-and-a-half awaiting the arrival of my soon-to-be colleagues from Berkeley. During that time I lived like a desert hermit: I ate little and alone, took walks by myself, talked to no one, retired early. I was just too weary and too sad to do otherwise. But unlike a desert hermit, devastating illness, disfiguring surgery and pending divorce were finally beginning to take their toll. Too much had happened too fast.

I tried to catch up on "Being Time"—not doing, not working, accomplishing, meeting deadlines nor even trying to pretend to be strong. Just being . . . being alone.

What a way to begin the New Year . . .

Survival Rule #5:

Build your own support group right away—family members, friends, therapists, clergy, co-workers, male and female—for it will be their love and their care that will give you strength for the battles, so that you may win your war. How do you do this? Simply ask them.

VI

WOLFGANG

"The wise man's teaching is a life-giving fountain,
for eluding the snares of death."
Proverbs 13:14
The Jerusalem Bible

Montreal and Dorion, Quebec—

Wolfgang Luthe burst through the front door in a flurry of snow and controlled energy. I found him to be aloof, exacting and total humorless—almost arrogant and stereotypically German—or so he seemed at first. All he needed to complete the perfect film caricature would be to look through a monocle and smoke cigarettes European-style.

Each afternoon he would ski about a half-mile from his small country house by the frozen Lake of Two Mountains to the two-story French provincial house across the road where my California classmates, Gina and Marge, and I were staying. Both houses were located outside the little village of Dorion, just north of Montreal.

Precisely at four o'clock, Dr. Luthe entered the hall. In a most formal fashion, he would nod and greet us. Then he'd pull off his black gloves and neck scarf, stomp the snow from his boots and brush his black ski suit—all done with precise vigor—and carefully place everything in the furnace room to dry. Only then would class begin.

I'll forever remember that first session. Dr. Luthe seemed to me at once the classic Old World German professor and a Tibetan guru. In reality, he was a medical doctor, psychoanalyst and one of the world's leading authorities on split-brain research—the study of the division of labor between right and left hemispheres of the brain—the basis of this course I'd come all those miles to learn.

For several interminable hours that afternoon, Luthe sat seemingly immobile on a natural goatskin rug spread across a highly-polished handmade wooden bench, one he himself had made and polished, as he had all the other furniture. His slightly graying, baby-fine copper-colored hair and his smooth ruddy complexion defied an age category. So did his clothes. That day, and every day, he wore soft fawn or dove-gray corduroy pants and checkered shirts of red- or blue-and white. Ankles crossed, he seemed motionless as he puffed serenely and endlessly on American cigarettes, Lucky Strikes, in a decidedly European fashion. Occasionally he tilted back his head to better peer at us, not through a monocle, but through black horn-rimmed, half-glasses perched on the end of a rather aristocratic-looking nose. Each time he looked at me, I felt as though he were looking through me and maybe several generations before me.

"Why do you want to take this course?" he asked abruptly.

My stock answer of wanting to find a line of work that offered longer-lasting satisfaction than newspapers and allowed closer work with people sounded, I thought, somewhat contrived. I think he thought so, too.

"What about your surgery?" he asked. "How are you feeling about that?"

"Oh, I've had a few bad moments," I answered, recalling the Reach for Recovery episode and my first confrontation between body, mirror and mind, "but never a bad day."

"You've never had a bad day?"

"No, I feel it's best not to dwell on it . . ." My good little patient's smile faded under his sober scrutiny.

"I see," was all he said. "What do you know about the Creativity Mobilization Technique?" he asked us all.

The other two knew a lot. They had in fact already begun the process known as "no-thought mess-painting" at home. I knew next to nothing. All I knew was the little I'd barely scanned in Fr. Tom's textbook (Luthe): tempera paints were used in abstract strokes brushed on newspapers, five stages of mental reactivity were experienced in the process. Somehow in each session, negative emotion would be discharged to permit the activation of creative, positive feelings.

Luthe explained this technique, his imperious manner mollified by his soft spoken-voice and charming German accent sprinkled liberally with "zeess" and "zat." The longer he talked, the more bizarre the whole process began to sound to me. I began to wonder what I'd gotten myself into.

"You are to keep a journal of your painting activities," Luthe continued.

Finally, I thought, a part I can understand. Journals are second nature to me.

"See what happens . . . Just follow instructions and see . . . You will learn surprising things about yourself. You should paint at least once a day . . . Use the remainder of your time to study the textbook. Each day at four o'clock, we'll start class and review the text along with all your paintings.

"Remember when you begin—you single most important instruction is to make a mess. In fact, you are to make the *biggest possible mess!*

"Good day. I will see you tomorrow at four. In the meantime, you have much to do to prepare for painting."

Then he methodically donned his ski suit and cap, his boots, scarf and gloves, stepped out into the wind and snow flurries and skied down the road to his little house on the edge of the frozen lake.

The three of us spent the rest of that January afternoon discussing that remarkable introductory CMT class and the even more remarkable Wolfgang. As we talked we worked, getting to know the painting room, equipment and our reasons for coming. Gina, an art therapist, was taking the course to use in her work with the aged in Berkeley. She'd met Luthe once before at a California seminar where he was lecturing. She said he was a genius.

Gina was very tall, about 5'11", and very thin, which only made her seem taller, and she was as calm as she was angular. She'd once been married to a famous artist whom she mentioned a lot, but whose name I could never recall.

Her friend Marge was a short, round, hyper housewife with cropped, wiry, dark-gray hair. She chain-smoked almost as unendingly as Luthe. Marge said she wanted to teach the course back home in Sausalito—where everything else in the world is taught, my skeptical side thought. I felt sure she was taking the course primarily because it was yet another adventure to share with Gina.

I told each of them I really wasn't sure why I was taking CMT.

Even though they were both "fifty-something" and I was thirty-five, we felt like schoolgirls as we cut, pasted and constructed lightweight styrofoam into stackable painting boards, and pared one-inch brushes to precisely 3/4-inch size, as per Luthe's instructions. Mixing tempra paints in one-pound coffee cans, I was in the first grade all over again. Eight vivid colors—red, blue, yellow, green, violet, brown, black and white—with yellow-handled brushes jutting from the cans looked intriguing. We were all anxious to begin first thing the next morning, as darkness had fallen all around us.

As I fell asleep that night, my thoughts flowed quietly and contentedly for the first time in a long, long time . . . '77 must be my year . . . a benign biopsy . . . and they've assured me that radiotherapy will take care of any errant cells. The long-pre-

pared for, long-overdue marital separation has finally begun . .
. and here I am in snow-bound Canada, hundreds of miles
from pain and problems . . . it's so cold here, if I can't solve my
problems, maybe I could just freeze them a while . . . ready to
start a whole, new creative career . . . Life looks up. I wondered
what my son was doing back in Texas and what kind of winter's day this had been in Arizona . . . smiling at the thought of
telling my cowboy-father about this strange painting process
creating the "biggest possible mess . . ."

Dreaming of a brand new beginning as new snow began
falling . . . God, how I wanted to be brand new . . .

Survival Rule #6:

To guide you through this new, unchartered territory, buy two paperback books immediately—*Getting Well Again*, by O. Carl Simonton, M.D., and Stephanie Matthews-Simonton, the best step-by-step course through the challenge of cancer back to health, and *How to Survive the Loss of a Love*, by Colgrove, Bloomfield and McWilliams, a survival guide for the loss of anything—especially health.

VII

TRUE COLORS

"In the deserts of the heart
Let the healing fountain start . . ."
"In Memory of W.B. Yeats"
W. H. Auden

The next morning I was the first scheduled to paint. I didn't have the slightest idea what to expect. Carefully making my way down the steep and slippery stairs from my bedroom at seven, my notebook on one hand and a blue and white kerchief in the other to protect my hair from spattering paint, I felt much like a schoolgirl in a foreign exchange program. Instead of rushing into the painting room, I wished I could just linger over a cup of coffee or two and visit with Gina and Marge. This was somehow evolving into much too structured a routine for my taste.

After only one cup of coffee, however, I tied my kerchief around my hair, entered the painting room and shut the door. I sat down on the three-legged stool in the corner and opened my notebook. For the longest time I could think of nothing to write. I just sat and gazed out the window at the snow and then at the painting table, then back to the snow. Finally I simply described what I saw and how it made me feel:

"The White Threshold": The snow continues to fall and I'm about to begin. The messy paint cans stand neatly in a row—their yellow tongues taunting me to start. Despite heady, dizzy apprehension, I cannot stop smiling about the "New Beginning." First a deep sigh, and now the confrontation with color and black and white to paint away the pain . . .

In one session, my emotions ran the complete gamut of possibilities. Surprisingly, anger and rage seemed to predominate, expressed in slashes of fiery red and splashes of black, the color I usually abhor. It has always represented tome (in things, not people) evil, sickness, pain and death, and I was astonished to find myself turning in the black brush over and over. There were tears two or three times. Then suddenly an explicable sensation of calm, bordering on bewilderment.

Afterward, I climbed the narrow, crooked stairs, even more slippery since removing my paint-spattered tennis shoes, and settled down to fill in all the sensation-describing charts Luthe gave us and to write in my journal.

I felt numb as I slipped into a hot bubble bath in the antique footed tub. I tried to sort through emotions while methodically going through all the after-motions, my naked body rising repeatedly out of the water to gaze again and again through the window above the tub at the vast whiteness of snow and ice on trees and road and the Lake of Two Mountains.

In the days that followed apprehension gave way to anticipation. I could see only good coming from the experience of breaking through emotional shells. The second day I painted, I felt just like a little girl again—I slathered paint across the pages, delighted to have permission to make such a mess. I began whistling and felt such elation that I burst into a childhood nonsense song—

*"With a knick-knack paddy-whack, give a dog a bone,
This old man came rolling home . . ."*

Throughout the session I felt the joy and eagerness of new beginnings. And the painting so heightened my sense of color, that while pushing a grocery cart in Dorion later that afternoon I was overwhelmed by the ordinary display of prosaic products—rows and rows of colored paper towels and tissues and toilet paper and baby items. All the yellows, pinks, greens, blues and lavenders had become for me a veritable shimmering fantasia. That's when I understood what Luthe meant by "receptivity."

All was seemingly going well. But as the week progressed, my painting sessions began to bring more and more emotional pain to the surface. I became correspondingly more tired—and irritable. I was unduly short with Marge and Gina the next time we drove into Dorion. My only consolation was that Morris was home when I called. We talked only a short while, and I don't really remember the subject matter. But I remember how far away I seemed from everyone I loved. And I recall that upon our return to the Lake of Two Mountains, my resistance went up—or crashed down—like a fortress gate, forming my soul's last bastion of stubborn defiance, a barbed-wire-wrapped barricade impervious to any and all efforts to storm it.

Survival Rule #7:

Say a resounding "YES" to Life. Now more than ever be open to *new* ideas, methods of healing and wholeness. Explore *new* avenues to reach your goal—complete and vibrant wellness.

VIII

RED RAGE

"Grave men, near death, who see with blinding sight . . .
. . . Rage, rage against the dying of the light."
"Do Not Go Gentle Into That Good Night"

Dylan Thomas

Feelings of weary discontent grew stronger by morning. Over coffee, I grumbled to myself and to my journal. This daily diary—a simple three-ring notebook - became my confessor, my opiate, my guide. I learned much from it by reading what my soul poured onto its pages. And that morning I confessed, "I sure as hell don't feel like painting . . ."

I was always completely honest in my journal. It was for my eyes only then, but for anyone who can learn from it now. It's the only way to really know me. Its pages reveal experiences and emotions I could never reveal face-to-face in a conversation. I didn't even know they were part of me until Luthe's surprising process pulled them from my unconscious.

A friendly warning, however—these next entries are not filled with lighthearted musings. Instead these are howlings of an animal trapped, wounded in a tempest—keening cries and feeble mewlings—and sometimes just a silent, scream of terror.

My persistent fatigue was my final attempt to avoid what *I had to go through*—my spirits last relentless effort to run away, to burrow down and sleep for all eternity—while smiling and pretending "I've never had a bad day."

Luthe said nothing the first class period that I appeared with no paintings. The second night I arrived empty-handed, his quiet, but contemptuous anger turned his face into an icy sneer. His eyes blazed. He was livid, but still he said nothing. When Gina and Marge went to the kitchen to prepare tea for our break, he confronted me.

"Why didn't you paint?"

"I've just been too tired." I sounded whiny and sulky even to myself.

"Too tired?" he snorted. *"Too tired!* I'm trying to reach that part of you that is *slowly dying*—and you're too *tired?!* You'd better learn to cope, sister . . ."

I couldn't cope. Suddenly sorrow and fear overwhelmed me. My old "fight or flight" syndrome flared. I fled to my room.

My journal entries that night describe what ensued:

> *BEFORE: Sunday, 11 p.m.*
>
> *Did not paint at all yesterday—and I'm starting to paint very late tonight. I left the session with Dr. Luthe early and abruptly because I was too upset to stay in the group; I could not keep from crying uncontrollably.*
>
> *The power of words hit home again. His criticism of actions I feel is merited. But his words are deliberately designed to zero in on the "Mess" from a new perspective— words that cut quickly and cleanly and one is left confronting yet again another aspect of self or reality that wanted to stay undiscovered beneath the scars. But the scab is ripped off mercilessly and the stitches ripped open and one is left bleeding—again . . . He wanted to reach that part of me that is "slowly dying," he said. And the words "slowly dying" unleashed a veritable screaming zoo of ani-*

*mal emotions: rage at him, frustration and anger for put-
ting myself in such an intense, exhausting milieu now, when
I was hoping for a respite from tension and tiring, hope-
lessly demanding personal situations; anger—no, not
anger—RAGE and futile sadness of feeling trapped and
helpless for not being able to cope—again.*

*Learn to cope, baby—or "sister" as the doctor called
me—a term I consider as unkind as it is patronizing—"or
you're in for a lot of trouble."*

*Wouldn't it be gratifying—just once!—to be the one
who could cope and be all together and "in charge"?—not
only of one's emotions in any given situation, but of one's
body as well?*

*But once again, it's the "others" who are in charge, who
control themselves so precisely they hardly move, just a foot
twisting slowly, occasionally, to ruin the picture of perfect
repose and self-satisfaction, and it is I who run, this time to
my room to let the tears really and finally begin. At first only
blinding me, then streaming down my face, undammed tears
soon turned into shuddering sobs I tried to smother in the
pillow I was pounding with my fists.*

*I suddenly realized the best thing would be to paint. I
wanted to start immediately, but could still hear the others
in the session. What is it about group dynamics that causes
remaining members of a group to draw closer together and
cooperate and act ingratiatingly one toward the other when
one of the group bolts or is chastised by the master? I'm as
guilty as anyone. Are we all so damned eager to please that
we will do or say anything to gain favor? The laughter I
hear only depresses me, or should I say disgusts me, when I
hear it between my own gasps of crying . . .*

I heard the front door shut, signaling Luthe's departure,
and I stumbled down the stairs to paint—sobbing, trembling,
slamming doors and equipment around, only to discover most

of the paint was dry. I unleashed some of my rage on the big cans of powdered tempra, slamming them down on the table, hitting the lids with the screwdriver, shoving my hand into the can and grabbing fistfuls of messy powder. I flung the powdery colors into the mixing cans, dashing a cup of water into the mess and jabbed at the mixture with the brushes—all the while weeping, sobbing, shaking and throwing things.

The red paint can was last and completely dry. When I threw water onto the handful of vivid red powder, it turned instantly to blood and pain.

I shouted "No! No!" and bent over double, violently, as though someone had hit me with tremendous force in the stomach. Trembling so I could hardly stand, I barely managed to pull myself upright only to be hit with wave upon wave of nausea and dizziness. Each time I saw the red paint, my head jerked violently to the left two or three times, not wanting to see, wanting to look at anything but the "blood." My hands shook fiercely and my sobs grew louder, more body-rending. At times I stomped my feet and shook my head in horror at the "blood" and the "pain" that slashed across the page—and the word "dying" kept sounding endlessly in my head.

I kept moaning the words "blood" and "pain" and "dying"—and my horror at seeing the "blood" splashing brought visions of blood spewing from my mouth after the last surgery. "A little too much anesthesia sometimes causes this reaction," the nurse explained, as I kept vomiting and coughing blood and blood and more blood . . . "You've lost an awful lot of blood," the doctor told me after the second operation, "that's why you fainted." Is this what it's like to die?—the blackness, the void, the nothingness, just the initial ringing in the ears.

Black death, black cancer slashed across the red—death and cancer and rage at not being in control of *even my own body*.

Then with the death, the funeral . . . Remember the cavernous room filled with caskets while doing research for the articles on funerals? The lavenders of mourning started mixing with the reds and blacks of bleeding and dying.

And then remember the test on "Attitudes Toward Death" from that university professor?—"You're not afraid of death," he explained in a pale gray tomb-line room, "but of painful and prolonged illness." And then a month later, I learned the "painful and prolonged illness" was here . . . The benign little lump they said "would go away all by itself" was not benign and was no longer little.

So then it's others who take charge of your body—this one to take blood, lots of blood, for lots of test—*How many times?!!* Don't take too much, I already lost enough, the doctor said. "Can't give you blood, you see, because the lymph nodes are gone and the risk of infection is too great . . .

My rage and frustration continued. Then just as I was beginning to feel a little less frantic and my crying subsided somewhat, I picked up the newspaper page with a series of photographs of a woman checking her bare breasts for cancer. The headline read: "La Corps de Femme"—The Woman's Body . . .

My God—how macabre! I'd been hit again. More nausea, more pain, my head hurting terribly . . . My God, I guess I need to cry even more . . . I carried the paper by the corner with my fingertips, trembling and shuddering at the bitter irony of this happening. This time I was so sickened by the red gore spilling across the two—*think of it, two!*—healthy breasts that the painting strokes became long and slow and horrible.

I did not cover all the photos. They were too fascinating. But the red brush came up again and again, then some black strokes for the cancer spreading, and then more blood and pain. I finished and set it slowly and carefully on the stack of the other "barbouillages" and continued painting and weeping . . . which soon diminished . . . only to pick up another page exactly like the other—- the rows of photos of the bare-breast-ed woman. I started to slash red on it, then I took a deep breath, stepped back and decided to set it aside for an experimental painting at the end.

I completed several more mess-paintings, experimented with "La Corps de Femme" page, then stopped. Feeling considerable unburdened and somewhat relaxed, although not nearly as much as I should, I wanted to go to bed. My mind and my body craved sleep. However, I made what I consider to be a grave error—I slowly removed my paintings from the room—one by one—studying each as I carried it, from the last to the first, and stacked them in their drying trays. By so doing, I relived the whole experience.

Afterwards, it looked as though a butchering orgy had taken place. Red was splashed everywhere—walls, floor, table, windows. I started to clean it up, but the red started smearing and I started crying and shaking . . . Had to leave the mess.

Then it was time to soak in the ancient tub and once again confront the body that no longer looks like the woman in those photographs.

Much later, my head hurt and I felt exhausted, depleted after writing and filling out all Luthe's charts. It's obvious I either didn't paint long enough or the automatic reviewing of the paintings when I removed them from the room opened the floodgates again.

I'm astonished, I wrote in my journal, at what happened in there tonight. First, by the synchronicity of those newspapers appearing—- being printed that very day—precisely when I needed to break through such pent up pain. And secondly, I'm amazed by the passionate explosion of that pain. I thought I had coped quite well with the medical situation, only to discover a red rage in this peaceful white countryside.

Survival Rule #8:

Anger, even rage, is a vital part of the recovery process. Allow the anger to rise, to spew out, so that it does not stay seething within, blocking the healing process. Your system needs all the equilibrium and strength it can find to heal you.

Deal with rage in productive ways. In the CMT process, one learns that the combination of large muscle movements and verbalizing is most conducive in neutralizing stress; i.e., long, stomping, curse-darn-swearing walks, throwing cheap dishes at a rock wall while voicing your anger.

Therapy—many kinds of therapy are good—art, dance, music therapy—and sometimes it's helpful to simply be alone and write out your pain and frustration about being betrayed by your own body. The CMT process proved most successful for me; up to that point it was the only acceptable place to vent my anger.

Whatever you do, DON'T SUFFER IN ANGELIC SILENCE. MARTYRS DO NOT SURVIVE.

IX

STORM

"The ice was here, the ice was there,
The ice was all around;
It cracked and growled, and roared and howled . . .
. . . And I had done a hellish thing . . .:
"The Rime of the Ancient Mariner"
Samuel Taylor Coleridge

By nightfall, the whine of the wind grew louder and wilder, developing into shrieks and cries in the dark. By morning the biggest blizzard in the record of a hundred years lashed Montreal and its environs. We could not even see the lake across the road for the fury of the snow. The screeching wind whipped power poles to and fro—their connecting lines sagged impotently in several places visible from our windows. When the lights began to blink off and on, Gina suggested w should mark chairs and benches that could burn the most readily in the standby woodburning stove in case of power failure. This was perhaps our most desperate thought.

But the violence of the storm did not altogether frighten us. It was such an extraordinary reality—especially for me. How often does an Arizona desert woman experience a snowstorm, much less one of this grandeur and dimension? Nor did the thought of possible total isolation greatly trouble me. I felt certain we could survive. Maybe my ignorance of snow and sub-zero temperatures betrayed me, but so preoccupied was I with my inner storm, that even a blizzard of monumental proportions seemed tame by comparison.

The Arctic blast's noise level, however, did not help my physical condition. I stayed awake most of that night listening to the wind's awesome power, and the resultant weariness added greatly to my already acute battle fatigue and depression—consequences of breaking into long-locked chambers of distressing memories. No wonder my resistance had gone up so stubbornly. It was my soul's self-preservation system. Alarm bells were ringing, clanging loudly, warning what painful territory I was about to explore. But this time, I had to ignore the tolling. It was time to *face* the pain, go *through* it, get on the other side of it—not circumvent it as in all the years past—not if I wanted to survive.

The storm did not keep us from our schedule. If anything we concentrated more determinedly, studying and painting with more fervor in order to escape feeling overwhelmed by the wrath of the tempest.

I was the last to paint that morning, and once I started, so engrossing was the session I forgot the storm outside. To this day I cannot read the following journal entry without weeping. It brings to the surface a subject I spent nineteen years trying to bury: pushing it back, denying it, closing my eyes, running away. Now, in this place, locked in by Mother Nature herself, I had no place else to run . . .

JOURNAL ENTRIES:

> *BEFORE: Exhaustion, depression, headache, knots in stomach, nerves strung out from lack of sleep . . . As I mix the paints, I listen to the howling of the wind and wonder. .*

DURING: Years of sorrow turned into colors and strokes across the pages . . . focusing on my mother . . . missing her, but especially remembering her battle with cancer. Operation after operation—the last one, brain surgery, to keep her from experiencing any pain—anymore. I can still vividly see the hideous loops of dried blood, looking like big black stitches framing her face where the folds of flesh were brought together and in places overlapped . . . Lose your children, lose your meaning for living, lose body parts, lose your life . . . Nineteen years ago and how much greater her terror and pain must have been.

Separated from her while still an infant, I was finally reunited with her one year before she died. By that time she had already suffered two radical mastectomies, a hysterectomy, a spinal operation. Chemotherapy had ravaged her hair and therapeutic testosterone had deepened her voice and sprouted a bearded growth on her chin and upper lip. This beautiful, loving, warm woman had become someone, some thing I didn't even recognize. I knew she was dying and I was so afraid of being near her—the sickness, the metal walker she had to use and the dying terrified me . . .

After yearning to be near her all my life, when it finally happened, I was afraid.

She was very brave and never spoke of the terrible pain—and I did not know until this instant, writing this, that I was trying to live up to her model of courage and selflessness. It killed her and I am left knowing that when I had the chance, I didn't help her, did not become close to her. The guilt and pain from that failure suffocate me. 'And I have done a hellish thing . . .'

I painted her funeral and death in lavenders and blacks and attacked the cancer and the bleeding with slashes of red—all the while crying inconsolably, moaning and stroking my head and my side with my free hand. My tears of sorrow spilled into the paint, and through the dizziness

and nausea and the gasping for air that followed, I reliv-
ed both her fear and mine.
    The painting strokes were generally long and slow,
and soon I began to breathe easily again, and so did peace
and understanding.

    AFTER: Later, after a hot bath, I felt a deep quietness
and a sense of healing and renewal. This feeling was so
intense I decided to wear a new pair of shoes that I'd been
saving for a special occasion . . .

In class that night under Luthe's bright light, the soft hue of violet in my paintings once again became the exact color of my mother's linen suit as she lay in her casket. Just as in my first breakthrough session, when the red paint became "blood," the black paint, "cancer cells," now violet became my mother's funeral shroud. I thought I had forgotten. But that soul-piercing sorrowful memory had been merely locked away, waiting for the healing key—a simple can of paint and a 3/4 inch paintbrush.

Nineteen years is a long time to hold back mourning.

My sorrow, my tears were not the only signs of healing. In the midst of this grieving session, my free hand stroked my head and body as I painted, as I cried. Luthe explained this to me: Because I was not near my mother, even as an infant, I missed a mother's nurturing, tender stroking. I was not consciously aware of this, but my unconscious had not forgotten. And this amazing process was automatically— *"autogenical-*
ly"—healing that memory.

The story spent itself. All that remained of the blizzard and its ragings was a blanket of soft, new snow—along with the 15- to 20-foot drifts in places where the snowplows had cut their paths. My own storm was spent, too, at least for a while. Luthe asked me to stay in Montreal—first of all, to continue, painting, to work through the grieving stage I'd entered, and secondly to work with him as editor and translator of his written work. But it was nearing time to return to Houston. And I was finally beginning to listen to what was inside me—I needed a break, a respite before painting again, in order to absorb, evaluate and adjust to what I'd learned since my "breakthrough." I know Dr. Luthe was sincerely afraid I might not continue painting, and were I to stop altogether, the results would have been disastrous. But I knew I would continue. I was convinced my life depended on it.

Marge was the first to leave. When departure came, I volunteered to drive her to the airport. Then the Gremlin and I explored Montreal—the city atop "Mount Royal."

One of my most outstanding memories of the city was my recurring surprise in the galleries on and near Jacques Cartier Square in Old Montreal—surprise not at the types of paintings I found, but at my preferences. Only those with great vitality, with vibrancy, with life, attracted me. Gone was my desire to gaze upon studied static forms. My eye was drawn again and again to the abstract, impressionistic flow of color. Rationalism had to be filled with energy or I lost immediate interest.

Each time I stepped out onto the sidewalks, the inside of my nostrils froze. The driving wind pierced my brain through the icy tunnels of my ears, and despite two pair of thermal longjohns, a pair of heavy pantyhose, two pair of knee-high wool socks, lined leather boots, lined wool pants, two sweaters, a heavy wool coat (made in Finland, for *their* winters), cashmere cap and muffler, two pair of woolen mittens, I experienced more sub-zero, heart-numbing cold than I'd ever dreamed possible. I didn't stop to window-shop. I dashed from gallery to boutique to gallery just for a few minutes of thawing.

Waiting for the little Gremlin's heater to warm up for the drive back to the Lake of Two Mountains, I remember shivering—great teeth-clattering shuddering might be more accurate—as I looked out at blue-silver-white barelimbed trees covered with snow and ice, and I counted more fur-coated persons bustling about than I had seen in my entire lifetime. For the first time, I coveted furs, full-length designs in mink, ermine, fox and even rabbit. But it was not their beauty I longed for, it was their warmth.

What I remember even more intensely than the piercing cold, however, was losing myself in the magnificence of Notre Dame Cathedral. Its stained glass windows seemed luminous, startling, primarily because of the sharp contrast of their crystalline reds and greens and cobalt blues to the expanse of gray stone inside and out, but also because of my own heightened receptivity to color.

I sat down on one of the back pews and stared all around. I knelt there, wanting, needing to feel close to God, to feel His presence. All I managed to feel was awe before the brilliant splendor of those windows of many colors. Awe and isolation, distance from God, *wherever* He was. And *whoever* this Great Spirit was, I didn't feel I knew Him at all. But just in case He could possibly be listening to this desert daughter who was so far off the path traveled by all these devout Quebecois surrounding me, I thanked Him for this extraordinary opportunity to discover the secrets of my soul.

Driving back to the little French house, gratitude still filled my thoughts. How long had I needed a place that allowed me to rage, to weep and mourn, to unburden my spirit—to be completely honest with myself, perhaps for the first time in all my thirty-five years. How thankful I felt that I could finally vent all my frustrations and fears, then recover and grow. Best of all, I could let it all pour out into the paint, not onto another man's soul.

Gina greeted me, glad to take a break from her studies for the CMT exam. Over steaming tea, she told me she'd decided to stay longer, to study at greater length with Luthe, "a chance in a lifetime," she said. And it would be, particularly since she'd experienced her own painting breakthrough while I was in the city—a session, she said, that had been triggered by my own.

As I changed into my painting clothes for the last time in the little house, I thought about how I would miss Gina. Each time I talked with her, I felt enriched, enlightened. What a good and equable companion she was. With a feeling of finality and sadness, I slowly tied my kerchief around my hair, picked up my notebook, and made my way down the narrow winding stairs. For "The Last Time Ever," I closed those doors, took my place on the little stool and began to write:

> *BEFORE: How tiny this room seems after the soaring heights of Notre Dame . . .*

> *DURING: "I want to live . . . I want to breathe . . . I want to live . . . let me breathe . . ." became my refrain during this entire painting session. I could not touch the heavy, hurting, suffocating colors of red, black and brown, but instead turned continuously to white, green and yellow, and only occasionally to blue and lavender. My thoughts centered on New Life, new chances, new beginnings . . . if only I could breathe. At times I was fighting so hard to get my breath I'd rise up on tiptoe to take in more air, to fill my lungs ever deeper. Not anguish, but hope, dominated my emotions, but it was hope of a desperate nature because I know there's not that much time left . . .*

> *AFTER: I looked at Gina's breakthrough paintings and listened to her readings from her journal. Then it was the sad time to drink one last cup of tea together and make plans for leaving the little French house on the Lake of Two Mountains.*
> *White prison—white liberation . . .*

Survival Rule #9:

Forgive yourself for "getting" cancer. Betrayal by one's own body is perhaps the ultimate—yet inevitable—treachery, but many factors entered into this medial equation. So be gentle with yourself. Nurture yourself and that spiritual side of you that will guide you to triumph.

X

OUTLAND

"... I wandered through the weird and lurid land-
scape of another planet ..."
"War of the Worlds"
Jeff Wayne's musical version

Montreal to Houston__

Happy to take a break from grueling classes, painting sessions and radiotherapy treatments, I went with friends to see
Sean Connery in "Outland." I love to watch Connery in anything 00 his expressive face can say more with a quirk of an
eyebrow than most actors can with their entire being.

"Outland," the alien environment of "Io," the third moon
of Jupiter appeared stark, cold, frightening and totally foreign—like hospitals. At the beginning of the film a worker
goes mad, a result of drug overdose. Panic-crazed, he runs into
an elevator that plunges him down, down, down into an
unpressurized zone, where, sans spacesuit, he explodes into
tiny fragments of what used to be a life.

Much to my bewilderment I started to shake, then I began
to weep. This scene seemed to be a metaphor for my life with
cancer. Each new cancer scare made me feel just like that—a

little more crazy. Each time, I felt more separated, isolated from "normal, healthy people," from Life, from God. Each new nodule became a closer encounter of terror. Each brought panic that made me want to run, that pulled me downward, spiraling into an abyss of wretchedness and desperation until I felt as though I, too, would explode—as though this epidermal suit of mine would disintegrate leaving nerves raw and bleeding, and I would shatter from the inside out.

I found myself on that dizzying, immobilizing Ionian elevator ride once again just as I began to feel strength and productive times returning. Despite extreme fatigue caused by all the weeks of radiotherapy, I'd worked enthusiastically, if sporadically, on plans for both private and group classes of CMT. Father Monahan compiled a list of former Omega Seminar students for my first group. He only needed a time, a definite date. I only needed Time—to gain a little more energy and a lot more confidence. Now it seems I'd need even more.

On March 2, 1977, only four months to the day after the modified radical surgery, and two and a half months after the last scare and biopsy, the nightmare returned. My journal recorded my emotional vertigo:

> *BEFORE: So the phone calls have stopped for a while. Morris went out with Alec and I'm alone. Now there's no further need to keep my voice steady, my expression smiling and calm. I'm alone with the heartbreak, the terror, the overwhelming disappointment and sorrow. This isn't like the last scare—the heaviness in my chest and the difficulties in swallowing and breathing which frightened me with nightmares of cancer coursing wildly through my chest. When Iglesias assured me that radiation had inflamed my esophagus, causing all the symptoms, I felt my life rise from limbo once again.*
>
> *Nor is this like the continual heaviness of heart whenever I feel the weight caused by loneliness and the conflict of*

separation and divorce. The failure of that part of my life creates an ongoing funeral dirge in my soul—a mournful, oppressive interior lament that plays over and over while the funeral drags on and vultures tear at the living flesh.

This latest dread, this terrorism striking treacherously from within is another tumor—this time in the breast itself. My one breast.

I rate myself a big "C" for "cheat." I've been cheating myself with the failure to give all of myself over to the healing process. I've allowed myself to be side-tracked a time after time—days I didn't paint, days I didn't center myself and use Simonton's healing imagery techniques, times I've allowed divorce problems and the resultant confusion and limbo to cloud my thinking, darken my emotions and tie my tongue with mind-numbing depression.

Now what, Sharon?

Now where? And when? How about now?!!

Do something for God's sake! For Christ's sake! For your own sake!

DURING: For ten paintings fear, sorrow poured out into the paints and onto the pages. For ten red and black horrors I felt desperation and unbelievable hopelessness—and then hope—that perhaps this new tumor is benign, hope that the cancer has not spread—and finally—hope that even if it has, I could still win.

Slowly, slowly, faith and courage began to displace the terror and the pain. During the despairing, I wept unceasingly and cried out over and over, "I've bled enough—Stop the bleeding—Stop the dying—Stop, oh, God, please stop the cancer."

An extraordinary panorama of my life passed through my mind in image after image in reverse chronological order. All the sorrows, fears, insecurities, anxieties—all the pain. And with those memories, the people who contributed to them came to mind. Then slowly somehow the images gave way to those who always seemed to alleviate the hurt—healing, soothing, loving people. What was it Maslow wrote about this?

I want time now, especially now that I've learned to live. I want to live with the fulfillment of my life's purpose, with joy and with love.

I'm asking for more time.

Is anyone listening?

Survival Rule #10:

Now is the time to eliminate as much "other stress" from your life as possible. Cancer is stress enough. "Other stress" includes disturbing situations, environments—even people. If annoying persons cannot be avoided, at least try to limit the amount of time spent with them. And if even this damage control is impossible, then greatly reward yourself later for your saintly patience in dealing with their particular poison.

One of the rewards might be to write about them in your journal and describe them in minute and exacting detailed caricature.

XI

ANNA

"I would I were alive again
To kiss the fingers of the rain,
To drink into my eyes the shine
Of every slanting silver line . . ."

"Renascence"

Edna St. Vincent Millay

By April Fool's Day, I felt like my old self again. God, I felt good!—rested, energetic, revved up to calm down and teach CMT. Only to Morris would I admit I also felt anxious, maybe even a little scared. Less than two weeks out of the hospital, I met the woman who was to be my first private student—she would also be my most challenging and rewarding teaching experience. Fr. Monahan had asked me to work with her.

"This may be her last chance," he told me. "She's dying of Hodgkin's disease."

Her name was Anna. She was too sick and weak to come to me, so I went to her. She met me at the door—a tall, big-boned woman, plainly dressed, wearing sensible, bone-colored lace-up shoes. I found it difficult to keep from staring in silent horror at her hair—iron-gray and shockingly short, less than a half-inch in length all over her head.

Oh, God, I thought, chemotherapy has taken its toll. I felt an immediate rush of compassion and pity for her. Then I'm ashamed to admit, I breathed gratitude—selfish gratitude that I'd been spared this terrible part of cancer's treatment. Just how terrible it must be was reflected in Anna's eyes—half-dead, glazed, I don't remember their true color. I only remember their hopeless despair clouded by a film of ever-present tears.

Anna was beaten. All she could do was sit in her rocking chair and weep. She couldn't even really talk—she just nodded or answered in monosyllables in response to any questions or comments. She managed to whisper only one complete sentence—"I haven't wanted to live since February."

That first hour and a half I learned Anna was fifty-six—a very old fifty-six—married and mother of six children, stair-stepped throughout their teenage years and early twenties. All but one still lived at home—six other people existed in her household and she felt estranged from each, believing they were all just waiting for her to die.

Her days consisted of resting in bed, taking oral chemotherapy daily, intravenous chemotherapy intermittently and being waited upon—and resented—by her family. She didn't cook, venture out of the house, read or even play music, despite being a serious musician all her life. Once a concert pianist, then a music teacher and director of music at her parish church, one of the largest in Houston, she had given it all up from lack of energy, lack of hope.

Friends, Anna found, as many cancer patients do, dwindle when you need them most. Fear of cancer becomes too threatening, particularly for those who have not come to terms with their *own* mortality. Cancer sometimes crushes even cherished friendships. And so with each new round of hospitalization and debilitating chemo, she had withdrawn more and more until finally, she felt completely isolated. Alone.

Deeply religious, Catholic, she believed her only solace

would be found in life after death.

After the first hour of this lopsided and saddening conversation, I realized Fr. Monahan was mistaken. This woman was not dying of Hodgkin's disease. She was dying of a broken spirit.

Everything I'd recently experienced seemed like child's play compared to Anna's sufferings. Once I got past her concentration-camp hair and started piercing together her story, I felt such empathy for this woman. I prayed I'd be able to make a difference in her life. I felt certain CMT could be the tool to reach her, if only, despite my reservations, she could muster enough energy to paint, or even shop for all the equipment and set up a painting room.

As I described the set-up and explained the process and written materials I'd brought to her, Anna just rocked and nodded. "Do you think you'd like to try this, Anna?"

She nodded while biting her lip and looking worried.

"Do you think you'll be able to handle it?" seriously doubting her success myself. "Anna, sometimes the painting can be quite strenuous," remembering some of my own sessions.

She nodded more determinedly, her eyes closed, her jaw set. I offered to shop for painting equipment for her. She shook her head. When I told her how this unusual painting technique had helped me overcome my own despair and panic, she crumbled in her chair and wept with heartwrenching, shuddering sobs, trying to believe, it seemed, that there could be a tiny shred of hope left in *this* life. I tried to comfort her, patting her shoulders, searching, searching for the right words of encouragement and understanding, handing her tissue after tissue. There was a sizable blue mound of them beside her rocking chair by the time she was calm and her tears once again came a silent, unending film across her eyes. When "class" ended and I leaned over to hug her good-bye, she clung to me like a brokenhearted child.

"No one," I told my father on the phone that night, "no one should have to die that alone, that unloved and miserable. Ever."

He cautioned me against expecting too much, fearing my disappointment. "Watch out ya don't turn this int' a crusade."

I assured him—and myself—I wasn't fooling myself into believing CMT could save her life. My goal was for her to start living, loving, enjoying whatever time she had left . . .

Survival Rule #11:

Get outside yourself. The fastest way to stop thinking about your fear, your pain, your misery is to talk to someone who is going through the same throes—or worse. Listen to them, help them in some way and do it often. Join a support group or simply look around the doctor's waiting room and *really see* the people there. Start a conversation. Life will surprise you with its comforting.

XII

IMAGES IN BLACK AND WHITE

"Made weak by time and fate, but strong in will
To strive, to seek, to find, and not to yield."
"Ulysses"
Alfred Lord Tennyson

My heart froze at the sight of him. I waited and watched from the doorway of his hospital room as Bernice Montcrief, chief of volunteers at Rosewood Hospital, entered to greet him. His name was Fred Black and even from a distance his visage was horrible to behold. A small white gauze bandage covered the hole left by his missing right eye. Growths hideous and huge protruded from his face and head and neck.

I couldn't breath. I felt sick. I wanted to run, but I was too scared to move.

Bernice called me and I forced my feet to move forward. I fervently prayed that revulsion would not show on my face, knowing full well that pity would show in my eyes. As I approached him, this piteous man with the dry mouth and the bristly thatch of straw-brown hair, the sight became even more cruel. The white bandage over his eye had slipped just under the overhanging socket of bone revealing a small, gaping hole through the bone in his forehead. Hard as I tried to keep from it, my eyes strayed upward. He noticed.

"That's where they had to go in again," he said, "to get the rest of it." The huge growths on his face and head were horrible egg-sized tumors worsened, aggravated into angry red by the seeds of radium implanted in their centers to kill the cancer burgeoning there.

He seemed not only glad I was there, but eager to tell me about his life.

"I used to be so strong," he told me. "All my life I've been a wrestler with so much strength and energy I could beat almost everybody." This was hard to imagine as he lay quietly in that barren hospital room barely able to lift his now-stringy arms, his hands cold as death as they clutched mine.

"It" started with the removal of his stomach which "really didn't bother me much at all," he said, "but when they had to remove my eye . . . I just couldn't take that.

"That became something I had to confront every day over and over—visible proof of how 'It' had spread." He paused for several long moments, remembering. "Depression and fear began to take over . . ." His voice caught and so did my breathing.

Fear and depression—how well I know their names. Old, old enemies of mine. Fear and Depression, I fight you every day now with few respites. And now after seeing the horror that they have wreaked upon this once strong and vibrant man, they've become stronger in my life.

Dr. Collins and Bernice want me to interview him, extract his life's story and the history of his illness. Do I have what it takes to go back? Can I return to his chamber of horrors? Will I be able to do the job, then come home and paint to vent my feelings of sorrow and fear? Is painting enough to dispel the brand of misery this experience generates in my already struggling soul? Can I do this for another human being who is suffering and most certainly dying, and for Dr. Collins, who is *always there* for men and women like Fred Black and me?

Or must I honestly admit that I cannot handle it? Should I confess that my survival depends upon concentrating only on positive experiences, that I cannot bear the terror of awakening in the middle of the night with this man's face hovering before me, feeling my own aches in wrists and legs and feet and back, wondering if "It" has spread inside me, too, only where it's not so horrible visible as it is in the pitiful, painful visage of Fred Black?

What is the answer?

The choice is mine. What am I made of?—certainly not of the same fibre as the Iglesias, Collinses and Montcriefs of the world. They're in the midst of this war because they choose to be. They've opted for the hard way, the path of the unsightly, heart-wrenching, sometimes hideous visions of suffering day after day. I'm in this war because my survival depends on it. That's not courage. It's stark terror.

"When in doubt, don't," my father always said. So for two days and nights I did nothing except agonize over my questionable capacity to once again confront Fred Black and his terrible cancers. Then just naturally and easily, in the course of a conversation with Morris I realized I not only could, but must. If I wanted to be able to live with myself, there would be no way to stay away.

Morris said, "Mom, this is a courageous thing you're doing."

"No, it's not courage," I told him, just as I told myself. "I'm scared witless. It's just something I have to do."

First, it would hurt Black too much to know that his appearance had repulsed me so much I couldn't return. Secondly, I would disappoint Dr. Collins. I want to do this as a labor of love for him; he's added so much strength and reassurance to my life. But most of all, I was surprised to learn, I want to do this for myself. I'm not *willing* to say "I'm not strong enough for this assignment." I Knew that if I would be working with other cancer patients through CMT, I'd face the problem again—or worse. I could hear Dr. Luthe: "You cannot conquer fear—or anything—by running from it . . . Face the tiger, Sharon!"

I faced him the next morning at ten. By concentrating on his good eye and his words and holding onto his dry icy hands, I was not so vividly aware of his tumors. By breathing deeply-and remembering what Mother Teresa once said in an interview about treating the dying as though you were treating Christ Himself—I overcame my nausea and my fear. I listened intently as he told me about his life—how as a child he'd been brutally abused by his father, how the angry child became an angry young man who grew older and angrier and held all his rage within him, his heart an ever-seething cauldron of roiling venom. Even his wrestling career was an attempt to channel and control his barely-beneath-the-surface wrath.

After a long pause he quietly said, "It's probably why I got sick in the first place."

Lying in that stark room, he said he deeply regretted wasting so much time on negative feelings of the past. I listened to his many memories, good and bad, and tried to make him smile occasionally, and just for an instant, I closed my eyes and tried to imagine my mother lying there, seeing her with the shorn scalp and loops of flesh and dried blood. With all my heart I wished I could have listened to her memories and made her smile.

It was good I faced the tiger. I learned much in that interview. Fred Black felt better for a short while, and longer I hope, but most important, I conquered my fear.

When I talked to Dr. Collins after the interview, he pointed out a rhyme, framed and hanging on his office wall:

> "A MAXIM FOR VIKINGS"
>> "Here is a fact
>>> that should help you to fight
>>>> a bit longer

> *"Things that don't act-*
> *ually kill you outright*
> *make you stronger."*

I do feel stronger.

"Strength is fleeting," I wrote in my journal. "Here I am—
only three weeks after conquering my terror of Fred Black—
and I'm a wreck. The threat of yet another biopsy creates pressures and tensions I'd forgotten. I can neither act calmly nor
think clearly. I jump at the slightest noise, cry at the slightest
provocation and lose my temper over inanities. Depression is
so devastating at this point, I wept all during lunch, choking
down an egg salad sandwich and a glass of milk for energy.
Actually I don't feel like eating anything.

I am *terrified* that this new growth is cancer. *More* cancer.
And if it is, where else has it spread?

To add to my terror, I saw a ghost at the clinic yesterday—
a ghost that haunts me, hounds my consciousness throughout
the day and awakens me at night.

A woman, about my age, was seated in a wheelchair in the
hallway attached to a chemotherapy hook-up. How beautiful
she was—and how sorrowful her green eyes. Swathed all in
hospital white, a white gown and robe with a white sheet over
her knees, white slippers, even her head was wrapped with a
white towel turban. Her pallor was such, even her skin seemed
merely a darker shade of white.

Obviously she was an in-patient and equally obvious was
the despair in her non-seeing eyes. She became hopelessness
personified to me.

The still white sight of her struck a blow to my stomach
and rib cage—full force—and left me trembling and gasping
for air and courage.

I saw myself in that chair.

I stared only for a moment, and then quickly slipped into
the ladies room behind her chair. I did not want her nor any-

one to see my panic.

"*God, do you HEAR me?*" I raged into the mirror in a whispered scream. "Do you *hear* me when I cry that *I DO NOT WANT* to end up in that chair?

"Are you *listening* to me?"

I gripped the sides of the sink to keep my buckling knees from completely giving way.

"I've just learned to *live*—" I wept.

"Merciful God—*Hear me*," I raged. "*I refuse to be in that chair!*"

Survival Rule #12:

When the desire to live burns with such intensity that your every thought, every word, your very breath and heartbeat become a prayer to God and the Universe for healing, then and only then will your meditations, visualizations and dreams become truly at One with all your medical procedures and you will know Wholeness.

XIII

GRAY LADY

"As though to breathe were life! . . .
. . . Come my friends.
'Tis not too late to seek a newer world . . .
. . . Tho' much is taken, much abides . . ."

"Ulysses"

Alfred Lord Tennyson

Daffodils and redbud trees bloomed profusely in the park across the street from our townhouse and all throughout the city and beyond. Wanting to enjoy their beauty at closer range, I took Sam and crossed the street to the park, hoping to soak in the sunshine before being soaked in paint. I took my notebook to write my first journal entry for the frightening week of the hospital return:

> BEFORE: It's early Sunday morning—my favorite time of the week, when the city and traffic stop their frenetic pace and all's quiet. This is the last weekend before my next surgery. Sam is with me, my constant, faithful companion. I watch him run and play as though he were a young beagle pup once again in his futile chase of a squirrel. This squirrel never tires of teasing and chiding Sam.

Something new catches his attention. It's the Gray Lady. She lives in the second townhouse in the second block. She walks her big, black scruffy poodle hesitantly, apologetically, as though she were sorry he's signing the shrubs and trees along the sidewalk. Occasionally she brushes back from her face a wisp of the gray hair that's escaped from her not-so-neat bun. Here potato-sack figure, which she's filled with perhaps far too many potatoes, seems to make her self-conscious as she moves heavily, ungracefully, down the sidewalk in her nondescript gray skirt and shapeless, colorless sweater. Her shoulders, curved into the question mark of her back and abdomen, seem permanently molded into the pressed-down slump of defeat and depression. Her once pretty face has eyes that seem to be non-seeing, just dully watching her dog go through his urgent motions. I wonder if her eyes are also gray, like the pallor of her skin. I cannot tell from here. She seems removed from the scene. Perhaps she's seen far too much pain to want to see anything anymore. She walks so listlessly, maybe she just learned she has cancer and is benumbed by fear. Or maybe she just has the flu and there's no one else to walk the poodle. More than likely, as most people I meet, she's simply not turned on to living.

She doesn't appear to see me—nor the glint of sunshine on the new blades of grass where I'm sitting, nor the cherry-pink profusion of blossoms on the redbud trees all around us. Not once does she raise her eyes to the clear, vivid blue sky. She doesn't even seem to notice the heavy perfume of blossoms permeating the air—even more remarkable now without weekday gasoline fumes disguising it.

The Gray Lady seems only half-alive.

I stop writing long enough to watch her and her big, black poodle pass by, forward and back, and disappear into the second townhouse and I wonder how long I've been like her—

half-alive, living only a limbo-like existence.

How long have we all been just like her? I want to say to my loved ones—What *are* you waiting for? Why in the name of God do you hesitate? Live life now! Love me *now*—don't wait until I'm dying. Cherish me this moment—not just when you see me slipping away. Relish my aliveness, my energy, my smile, as I do yours. Look into my eyes and truly *see* me, as I see you. Touch my hand, feel my warmth. And if you cannot celebrate my existence as I celebrate yours, at least salute the humanity in one, as the Navajo do. And I will salute you. Accept this meeting, this togetherness as a holy gift, for it is. Take *Time* for me and please understand—it is not so much that I'm afraid of dying as that I'm terrified of not truly living. Now that I've been so close to the edge of that final silence, that last separation and aloneness, I cannot bear being taken for granted.

Do you not realize that there is nothing, *no thing* more important than our Love for one another—not one more business meeting, not one more golf game, not even one more artistic creation—if it usurps the inestimable dignity, beauty and worth of Life, of one human being.

I cannot abide your slothful inattention. *See* me. *Hear* me. *Touch* me. Experience this Life spilling over in me, spilling out of my spirit with no one to see, hear or even notice.

Rejoice in this Life that burgeons within me, as I rejoice in yours, so that when the Light no longer shines through me, you will not bewail, "If only . . ."

> *I don't know why it took this threat of death to jolt me into Life?—to jar me into listening to distinct birds chirping, calling and answering each other, to nudge me into deeply inhaling the pungent fragrance of blossoms coming from everywhere in the neighborhood and awakening me to the new row of vivid daffodils at the far northeast corner of the park. They weren't there last week. Their strong, star-*

tling yellow has become for me the color of Hope—in my paintings and in my life. How bravely it contrasts with the gray of my despair.

Just a few more days now till I return to the hospital—again. What will it be this time? Health, Wholeness, Life and Joy? Or more cancer, terror, pain, sorrow and death? I'm opting for the former. Maybe if I paint often enough I can neutralize the fear and depression enough to bear this out with courage and faith and final victory . . .

DURING: Depression, lethargy and just trying to make it through the session.
Don't like the script—
Don't want to go back—
Maybe, just maybe, it might be for good news . . .

AFTER: Peace and optimism—again.
I'm running out of yellow paint.

One week later the news at the hospital was good—described in only one word—"benign." Before, I didn't know that "benign" meant "hope" and "peace" and "new beginnings." I have a friend named Alicia from Argentina whose medical history is parallel to my own, who likens the word "benign" to "Safe!"—"It's a split-second reaction," says Alicia. "You're stressed out, stretched out as far as you can possibly be without being torn completely in half, waiting, waiting waiting for the verdict, and when it comes—'Benign'—it's a pronouncement that you've won. You're safe. You're home."

For me, each time I heard that beautiful word, I felt it was an annunciation, a benediction, a blessing beyond the telling, and my world had to stop for a while to fully comprehend, to revel in how all the fear, all the sorrow that so froze the heart, the mind, are now transformed, melting into warm rivulets of lifegiving Joy.

Now instead of a wounding second mastectomy, I'm experiencing hoe that my life will start down a more positive, productive path. I'm feeling peace that could be defined as simply the absence of terror and panic. New beginnings are stirring within me—beginnings of confidence, of health, or striving, beginnings of faith and trust.

But most of all, Dear God, I'm filled with thanksgiving . . .

Survival Rule #13:

When you can turn and thank God for the graces coming into your life, not only *in spite of* what you are going through, but *because* of it, this is a great and healing "Yes! Yes! Yes!" response to Life.

XIV

TERROR

I am utterly spent and crushed;
I groan because of the tumult of my heart.
Psalms 38:8
Oxford Annotated Bible
For the thing which I greatly feared is come upon me,
and that which I was afraid of is come into me.
Job 3:25
Holy Bible King James Version

I thought I had escaped it. Chemotherapy. The thought sickens as well as terrifies me. Chemicals injected into my veins. I will be extremely sick, nauseated and weak the bearded chemotherapist told me. Not for him the doling out medicine by teaspoonfuls. He threw it at me a barrel-load at a time.

He stood before me, a Latin Peter Ustinov in a three piece suit and a black beard—only taller, handsomer and very intense. From a distance he'd always seemed gravely serious and maybe a trifle arrogant, maybe because I'd never seen him smile. Up close he seemed even more serious, but there was not a trace of arrogance, only concern and total candor. I bombarded him with questions and he shot back answers in his Peruvian accent and with every straight-arrow response I saw more clearly the only path left to me.

"Will I lose some or all of my long, dark-brown, super Shirley Temple curls?" I asked him, regretting the unfortunate analogy the minute the words were out of my mouth, considering her bilateral mastectomies.

"All of it."

"Will I become thin and haggard and drawn looking as so many I've seen?"

"Not necessarily thin—but haggard and drawn? Eventually, yes."

"How long will I have to take it?"

"Two full years—and you will get progressively weaker."

"Couldn't I just start on a super-vitamin and nutrition program and use imagery techniques and forego chemotherapy?"

"Absolutely not. You can do all those other things, but you cannot eliminate chemotherapy—especially with your family history." Then he described how breast cancer metastasizes—to the bone, the brain, the liver and the lungs.

Exactly my mother's scenario, I thought.

"But since they caught mine early, wouldn't my case be different?"

"From the size of the tumor they took from your breast, it is clear it had been there a long time."

"No more questions."

Abject terror engulfed me, interfered with my breathing—fear of more cancer, more pain, burning in the veins. My new challenge, it seems, will be to keep calm and steady and good-humored while they inject my body with God-knows-what kind of poison. "Systemic treatment" it's called, but it's spelled "T-E-R-R-O-R."

The only clear thoughts I took from that session were those of dying. Must death *always* hover?

I stopped at Sambo's coffee shop once again—not wanting to be alone, not willing to burden friends and family with the news just yet. I slowly sipped cup after cup of steaming coffee, trying not to think of Anna's concentration-camp hair, staring mostly at the incessant traffic and watching the endless stream of people coming and going through the double doors of the coffee shop, not really seeing any of them—until I saw her.

Long and lean and feline, she sauntered through the coffee shop in her tightly molded blue-jeans and her clinging oyster-shell tank top with its swooping, plunging neckline. All eyes, including mine, turned toward her and followed her every move. Heartbreakingly, I realized what made her appear so beautiful, so self-confidently sensual—her long, long, luxuri-ant lioness' mane of tawny hair.

Down her back it tumbled, thick and shining and glori-ous—and the realization I would soon be totally bald struck full force. My practiced calm crumbled. My mid-section began to tremble. My teeth began to chatter and my cup clattered in its saucer each time I tried to set it down, even using both hands. And for the first time throughout this whole medical ordeal I heard myself muttering over and over, "It's not fair . . ."

The thought of strolling lean and sensuously through any room in the world—bald—seemed ludicrous: the world had not yet heard of Sinead O'Connor and her audacity. And, I wondered, with my hair, will my femininity leave? bald is such a masculine word. What if the wig that I'll be fortunate enough to buy slips off in public?—leaving me more shorn than Delila's victim—cruelly deprived not only of strength, but of dignity and self-confidence as well? Will I become an object of derision and sport? I've seen how people scorn those whose hair has just started growing in—pointing, laughing at the strange, extreme hairdo. If they only knew what these peo-ple have endured—rather than an object of ridicule, their shorn scalp would be a crowning laurel of great courage.

Why is this harder for me, to accept the loss of hair more than the loss of part of my body? The hair will grow back. Is it because I remember the ages-old nightmare of my mother beckoning to me from the grave, with only a hank of thin, wispy hair hanging from her almost totally smooth scalp? The horror of it happening to me begins again, relentlessly.

Will they find cancer in the bone marrow?—in the axilla, the other breast? Are all these lymph nodes swollen because cancer has already manifested its "aggressiveness" in yet another young woman? Percentages—one after another were quoted to me regarding chances of reoccurrence, chances of recovery and total cure . . .

I want to be *more than another statistic*. I want to *beat* the percentages. I've never been a gambler and I've seen the ravaged beauty of my mother: her voice deepened, the bearded growth on her chin from all the male hormones, both breasts removed, all female organs extracted, vertebrae disintegrated, and finally, the brain surgery, with the shorn and shaven scalp and the horrible black loops of dried blood along the skin flap showing beneath the ugly stocking cap they later pulled over her poor suffering head.

I have seen your devastation, cancer, and I'm willing to go through the horror of having my hair come out by the handfuls, or brushfuls, in order to keep you from taking my body—organ by organ, cell by cell.

And so I will have my hair shorn very short *before* the adriamycin strikes. Not for me the waiting passively. I am not intimidated yet . . . and yet . . . "You are beautiful," I've been told a time or two. But it has always been more important to me to be beautiful *inside*. Now is the test. With the disappearance of outer beauty, will inner beauty become invisible because the outer vision is too horrible to behold?

I pray this is not so. I pray that enough Light will still shine so that I may still be effective for others. If I cannot, there is no reason to keep up the fight. Working with others has become the main reason for my existence. If I see pity, loathing or revulsion in their eyes, or God help me, in the eyes of my loved ones, I no longer would want to stay . . .

Through chattering teeth, I managed to say the word aloud to myself—"Chemotherapy."

How could this catch me so by surprise? I thought they'd promised. I was *sure* I'd heard them promise. But in truth what I'd heard was what I'd wanted, needed to hear. This was why Dr. Collins wanted me to keep in such close touch after radiotherapy; this was why that bearded chemotherapist looked at me so intently; this was why Iglesias wanted me to gain weight. I kept telling myself it was because he was Latin and liked women to be Botticelli beauties. They each had known all along. But two of them were giving me my medicine by teaspoonfuls, hoping I wouldn't find the taste to bitter a little at a time.

I took comfort once again from carrot cake and milk, knowing full well it would take much, much more to find courage for the months, years ahead.

Just at that moment, a Lincoln Continental, silver-gray like my dad's, drove through the parking lot. On the back window was a sticker that read, "God keeps his promises with rainbows." I decided to take comfort whenever and whenever I could and wrote the words down on a paper napkin. I later copied the words into my journal, but I carried that folded napkin with its promising words for months afterward.

Survival Rule #14:

Remember Luthe's words—

"You must face the tiger."

XV

FORT APACHE COURAGE

Ask, and it shall be given you; seek, and ye shall find;
knock, and it shall be opened unto you . . .
                                              Matthew 7:7
                            Holy Bible, King James Version

The Tucson Desert—

What is it about the desert that soothes my soul? Especially the Tucson desert with all its mountains surrounding—the immensity of the rugged Santa Catalinas to the north, the smooth, peaceful slopes of the Rincon range to the east, and to the west, the close and friendly Tucson Mountains burgeoning with saguaro, cat's claw and ocotillo. I love to breathe in this rough desert's vitality with its smell of mesquite.

I'd come to the desert once again to see my wise and witty cowboy father to tell him in person about chemotherapy, to soften the blow. Or so I told Morris—and myself. Looking back, I think I just needed a refresher course in courage. I got it—from the desert mountains and from the man.

My father matches the land—roughhewn, untamed, belonging to another era, enduring—no matter how much progress and Yankee development try to transform each. His

Code of the West is not that portrayed by Louis L'Amour with what my dad once described as "modern day counterfeit old time dime novels," nor, God forbid, that of the Spanish novelist, Camilo Jose Cela. It would be Cormac McCarthy and Larry McMurtry who would create a West true to the memories my father gave me, how it really used to be. McMurtry created two characters who seemed to flesh out the two alter egos of my father—Augustus McRae and Capt. Woodrow Call of *Lonesome Dove.* My father was as witty, compassionate and philosophical as Gus, and as stubborn a loner as Captain Call—and, I should add, as passionate in fury when pushed too far. Those two characters even used some of the same expressions and the same rhythm in their speech as my Dad.

On the plane I thought about how he sounded on the phone. I could tell he thought I was going to die. He grew up in a generation that thought a cancer verdict meant an irrevocable death sentence. How could he believe otherwise? Fearless about most things except for snakes—any kind of snake—he was the only person involved in this cancer ordeal more terrified than I. Yet from the beginning he talked to me of courage, especially my great-grandmother's variety, and he always tried to make me laugh.

I couldn't help but think of all the advice he'd given me throughout the years, some of it funny, all of it sage. I thought again about one of his favorite sayings, "There ain't any of us gettin' outta this alive . . ." He didn't say it anymore.

He always smiled proudly, beamingly each time he saw me, and despite the last-time-everness of his first look when we met at the Tucson airport that April afternoon, he still beamed helplessly. That alone reassured me. Everything about my father on that visit conveyed great strength to me, as always. What comfort I took from the absolute steadiness of his smiling, brown-eyed glaze, the stubborn, jutting set of his jaw, his massive shoulders and arms as he hugged me hello and patted me on the back with all the power and grace of a papa grizzly comforting his cub. Even his nose seemed invincible to me. Although it had been broken many times in his drinking, brawling youth, his was a grand nose of extraordinary character—strong, sharp, craggy with a slight hook at the bridge.

"Sure good t' see ya," he told me, his eyes shining.

He was dressed exactly as I'd known he'd be: cowboy shirt and western-cut pants, always in conservative earth tones, the wide soft leather belt with its sterling silver buckle inlaid zuni-style with a turquoise and coral thunderbird. He'd worn that same buckle for the last twenty years ever since he gave me his old silver one. And, of course, he was wearing a pair of custom-made cowboy boots. He owned over twenty pair of them. In his hand he carried his best straw Stetson of many X's. His garb never varied except for golf games, funerals and weddings, although when he gave me away as a bride of eighteen, he refused to wear a tuxedo and insisted instead upon his finest midnight blue western suit and black sharkskin boots, much to the chagrin of my one-time mother-in-law.

Despite his rough exterior, there's an indefinable quality about my father much like molten gold—pure, shining, malleable—a spiritual earthiness, or an earthy mysticism that priests recognized long before he let one sprinkle holy water on him. Each of them tried to draw him into the Catholic side of the Christian fold. One monsignor, who tried in vain to entice him from the golf course into mass on Sunday mornings, told him that he'd finally decided, in case of my father's untimely demise, to simply place Daddy's casket at the foot of the altar at St. Augustine Cathedral and instruct all the mourners to line up and throw golf balls at it.

I think this spiritual earthiness came from growing up at Fort Apache. Born in 1914 on my grandfather's ranch, he grew up close to the Apaches and at one with the land. God, how he loved the land, the ranch and his horses. Each time he talked about them, his eyes misted and there was an ever-present catch in his voice.

He came late to the big city, if you can call an over-sized cowtown like Tucson a big city—a cowboy of the old school with the old code of honor. His business slogan, taken from his high school year book, was "Ugly But Honest," but it isn't honest to call my father *ugly*. The word had a different, kinder connotation in those days. Rugged? Yes. Unpolished? In ball-room etiquette, perhaps. But ugly? Never. Make that gentle-manly macho, a by-product of his times. And kind. Aside from his wit, which I always hoped to inherit, loving kindness is my father's strongest trait.

"I've got a surprise for you in the trunk of the car," he told me as he carried my luggage out into the sunshine. He could-n't stop grinning. And he couldn't wait until we got home to give me his present. He never could wait to give presents. Even at Christmas we always celebrated early, my older brother Patrick and I opening gifts no later than six on Christmas Eve. My cowboy father claimed that Santa came first to our house because he and Santa knew each other personally—in fact, they were "compadres." He swore that each year in the fall, when he went on roundup to his friend's ranch in Colorado, the first thing all the cowpunchers did was round up Santa's reindeer before they even started looking for cattle.

"When ol' Santa comes to claim his fattened herd, why him and me, we always just sit around and shoot the bull for a while," he told us with that faraway smile of his. "No kid-din'," he always added for extra emphasis. I believed him, of course. My brother always smiled and winked at me.

The surprise?—a fine, *almost* new set of Ping golf clubs that he'd traded from a woman golf professional on tour. An old horse trader, if my father couldn't trade for something, he didn't want it. Carefully, almost reverently, he lifted a hand-some burnt orange leather bag from the trunk of his Continental. A complete set of Ping irons sparkled in the sun-shine alongside a full set of Power-Bilt woods with burnt-orange leather head covers.

At our favorite Mexican restaurant, the L&L, always our first stop when I returned home, he said, "Now I want you t' use those clubs ever' week and learn to hit *long*."

I knew what he was trying to say.

"Daddy, I'd like to, but there's a slight complication."

"Oh?" Always just "oh? when he thinks bad news is coming.

"I have to start chemotherapy."

"Really?" Pain filled his voice and his eyes. He began to pour billows of sugar into his iced tea. "For how long?"

"They tell me for two years."

He winced at the words.

"But," I quickly added, "it will keep the disease from spreading. I'm young so cells divide more quickly—they tell me the younger the person, the more aggressive the disease. Always "the disease." One didn't say the word "cancer" around my father.

His spoon attacked the mounds of sugar heaped at the bottom of his glass, vigorously, noisily, until other customers began to stare. Inspecting the white clouds rising in the brown liquid he asked almost apologetically, "I have to ask—will you lose your hair?"

"Yes, Daddy, I'm afraid so."

He stopped beating his iced tea, carefully placed the spoon down on his paper napkin and looked at me with such sorrow in his eyes my heart broke. "I'm real sorry to hear it, Sharon."

Then we both stared into our tea glasses, neither of us knowing what to say next, but I was remembering how beautiful he always thought my hair to be—enraged once at my one-time step-mother for applying an old-fashioned Lilt home wave to my already naturally curly tresses, turning them into the wild frizzies, and enraged twice when I cut it so short in my junior year in high school no curls could appear.

Our waitress brought our carne seca chimichangas amid much friendly waitress-type chatter, and we gratefully focused on the reality of dried beef, chile and flour tortillas.

"Excuse me just a minute," Daddy said. "You go ahead; I'll be right back."

He returned a few minutes later, his face pale and blotched, but gently smiling. He slid into the booth, took out his Buck pocket knife, and ignoring his chimichanga, cut a small, precise plug of Red Man tobacco and carefully placed it in his cheek.

"I want you t' remember just one thing," he said as he leaned back, "and I want you t' remember it as long as you live. Do you remember when you were little girl and things just weren't goin' right, you remember what I'd tell ya?—The sun don't shine on the same dog's back *ever'* day."

"I remember."

He leaned across the table and pounded his forefinger onto the surface with each word: "Well, by God, your turn's comin'! Anytime you start t' git down, you remember what I told you."

"I'll always remember, Daddy. I promise you."

He stared out the window for several minutes, then he looked at me and grinned as he carefully tucked the tobacco pouch back into his shirt pocket. "You know, Sharon, there's something I been meanin' to tell you about those clubs. I kinda wanted you to enjoy 'em awhile before I told you, but what the hell! I just made up that story about the woman pro—you'll be gettin' a bill from that young pro at Oro Valley any day now." His grin widened and his eyes sparkled from humor, and more, I suspect.

And with that, the subject of chemotherapy was closed. The rest of our time together we talked about everything under the sun except sickness: his Golf Game, for instance— he wasn't "playin' worth a fiddler's damn;" Favorite Books—he read voraciously, particularly history and biography, and he was in the midst of *The Patton Papers*; Politics—more conservative with each birthday, he swore he started out just a little to the right of Barry Goldwater; Movies (he never said "films") and Actors—if George C. Scott or Anthony Quinn starred in *anything*, he relished it, but as much as he cursed-darn-swore with "damn-it-to-hells," he hated movies filled with profanity. That subject always led to "The State of the World," and how, "by God, the world's goin' to hell faster'n a cuttin' horse after a maverick;" how it was just no longer like "the days of horse tradin' and cowpunchin' on the ranch" where if anybody cursed they had a reason.

Each homecoming proved the same. Whenever we were together we talked more than any two teenagers, and how we laughed!

I tried out my new clubs and played golf with him at Oro Valley where he introduced me to the "ruthless pro who'll sue if he doesn't get his money." Then we were off to the "fuhrer's party—"the fuhrer" being his close golfing friend and lawyer of German descent, 'who'll handle the pro's case for a substantial fee; he believes like I do, Sharon—you gotta make money off your friends and relatives."

Beneath the desert's silky, star-filled sky in the foothills of Tucson's Catalina Mountains, in the midst of dozens of people and the almost forgotten aroma of mesquite-broiled shrimp, my father, it seemed to me, was the most loved man there. Everyone wanted to be around Clyde and his humor. Frozen margaritas and beer flowed freely and so did raucous party laughter, all the men trying to out-punch-line the next, but my father was the hands-down funniest. Warmed up with black coffee only (a reformed alcoholic, he hadn't taken a drink in over twenty-nine years), he introduced me to everyone as his sister.

"My *older* sister," he clarified.

Then he launched into more of his favorite, funny tales of the ranch and all his cowpunchin' compadres." Deep affection was apparent in the continual ribbing between him and his friends, male and female of all ages. Many I'd known for years, but I enjoyed meeting new faces, especially Moore and Soleta. Each expressed mock shock and disbelief that I could possibly be my father's daughter— they each shook their head, "tsk-tsk-ing" as they looked from my features to my father's and back again. With perfectly sober expressions, each swore it to be genetically unlikely, if not downright impossible. Daddy feigned injury and I basked in the light of so much camaraderie. I nearly forgot about the coming ordeal.

A few days after my return to Houston, he sent me a letter in handwriting that ran off the page at a dreadful downhill slant:

Dear Sharon,

Like I told you on the phone, this golf pro is getting mighty nasty about his money. However, you made such an impression on "the fuhrer" that I'm sure he would defend you for nothing.

Also Moore and Soleta would gladly perjure themselves in your behalf. You are all Moore talks about—he also makes observations and comparisons to myself which don't please me at all, i.e., mixing babies, etc. He doesn't realize that after what he said to me it would only involve a $3 fine if I hung him.

I really hated to hear about the therapy. You have been superb to here, Sharon—just keep it up. Hope the closed will help with the wig.

All My Love,
Clyde

The enclosed was a most generous personal check—I could have bought a half-dozen Dolly Parton-like wigs if I'd wanted.

This short letter, one of three I'd received from him in my life, typified my cowboy-father. As always, with just a few words he heartened me. And he was as generous as he was kind. This givingness stemmed, I think, from stinging after-the-ranch memories of the depression that always haunted him—memories of owning only one or two shirts, one pair of pants, no money, no food and wearing holes in his one pair of shoes—he couldn't afford boots then. He never forgot anyone's generosity or kindness in those days and whenever failed to pass it on to others, whether through money, material goods, moral support and loyalty, or his gift of humor, the finest mask of Fort Apache courage.

Survival Rule #15:

Love is the Great and Unequaled Comforter. If you have no one who loves you with unconditional acceptance, find someone. They are there waiting for you—in your family, among your friends or acquaintances, in a support or prayer group. If, on assessment you realize you have no one, *get help fast.* Seek a counselor, priest, minister or psychologist and build from there.

If you still find no one who loves you, maybe you are not being lovable enough. Maybe you need to seek the second greatest comforter first—forgiveness. Forgive others. If you cannot find it in your heart to do it for them, do it for yourself. Without it there can be no true healing from within. Then forgive yourself. Forgiveness leads inevitably to Love.

Maybe you need the great unconditional lover—a dog—the best of all earthly examples of how to love and be loved.

XVI

COIFFED

What is sweeter than honey?
What is stronger than a lion?

Judges 14:18
Holy Bible King James Version

Houston to Huntsville—

Vanity, vanity—they name is surely Sharon. And because I am so vain, it took two and a half quaffs of my "poor-man's sangria" (grapefruit juice laced with burgundy wine) to numb me sufficiently to shampoo the tangles of my hair in the shower for the "Last-Time-Ever"—at least for a long time.

As the long tendrils trailed down my face, my back, my shoulders, the shampoo made it slick and sensuous. It would be very short that afternoon and gone completely within a week or two. The thought of losing my hair made me feel much like one preparing to enter the novitiate. That's only fitting. I am a novice at being bald. I couldn't help but think of Anna, her hair just beginning to grow out after her continued bouts with chemotherapy. It's probably a little over an inch long now—just one inch all over her head. Compared to Anna's sufferings of the past and present, I truly am a novice . . .

So traumatic would be this afternoon's shearing of my long, but short-lived locks, I would only entrust them to a friend who'd been cutting my hair since I moved to Texas. So I drove all the way from Houston to Huntsville for very personal TLC. I procrastinated with a side trip to the Huntsville Item. I sorely needed the nurturing and strength I always found among my compadres there, especially Rana and Michael. We opted for a long lunch of pizza and beer. Michael ordered sausage, mushroom and black olive knowing it was my favorite. Beer came by the pitcher, and after only one or two mugfuls, Michael began his "Did I ever tell you . . .?" stories, filled with knee-slapping, sometimes bawdy humor.

"Did I ever tell you about the two old cowpokes leanin' against a fence post watchin' a hefty, but tired lookin' bull?"

"No, Michael, you never did," Rana and I answered the stock response, whether he had or not. This time he hadn't.

Well, you see, said Michael, there was this rancher who had an old bull who just wasn't interested in cows anymore. He was just plumb wore out. And the rancher had just about given up on him.

'Y'know, I'm just gonna have to carry that ol' bull yonder to the feed lot. He just ain't performin'.'

'That's a durn shame,' said his friend, ''cause he's sure done real good fer ya fer many a year. Sown a lotta mighty fine calves. Before you give up on 'im why doncha have the vet take a look at 'im an' see if there's anythang he can do. Maybe he can put new life in the poor ol' thang.'

'Good idee,' said the owner of the bull, 'I'll do 'er.' And he did.

The next time the friend happened to drop by, he just couldn't believe his eyes. Frisky and feisty as a young calf, that same old bull was jumping on every cow in sight. He was mounting everything that moved and even jumped on a fence post or two. And in between 'jumpings' he'd race about and kick his heels. Darned if that ol' bull didn't look like he was smiling.

  'Well, I never would'a believed it,' the friend said, 'if I hadn't seen it with my own eyes. What happened?—Didja take 'im to the vet?'

  'Yup.'

  'Well, did he give 'im somethin'?'

  'Yup. Said it'd make him randy as a jackrabbit and jump everythin' but a mule.'

  'Well, what'd he give 'im?'

  'I dunno—but it tastes just like peppermint!'"

Michael just barely finished the word "peppermint" before Rana and I burst out laughing. I don't know if the story was that funny or we just badly needed to laugh but Rana and I both came apart at the punchline, especially me considering I'd just taken a big swig of beer. Michael, of course, kept a straight face, but he kept tugging on his mustache so we couldn't see him smile.

He had more "bull" stories to anesthetize me for the ordeal with the merciless edges of the scissors, but that one remained my favorite. It made me laugh all the way to the beauty shop. "Just like peppermint . . ." Oh, Lord . . . that's great! My dad would love that story."

I was still smiling as I walked up the sidewalk between two Rose of Sharon trees and started climbing the steps, but I still felt like a condemned prisoner walking "the last mile." Only my condemnation, my sentence will be "injection" not "the chair." Just like Ernest Benjamin Smith, (the young black man we all interviewed on Death Row on July 4, 1976 when the Supreme Court reinstated the death penalty). How much he and I have in common now I thought, including a shorn cap. Thinking of the interview with him the day room just outside Death Row at Ellis Unit, I stumbled and fell up the steps, crashing into the door of the shop.

Well, there's a first. Most people fall *down* steps. The only other person I knew who fell *up* stairs was my friend, Roberta, who's been accused of being my sister, only she's much shorter and much, much funnier. She fell up the steps of the Greyhound bus that would carry her away from home to college for the first time. As she tripped across the top step, she stumbled—*catapulted*, might be more accurate—across the aisle and slammed into the horrified bus driver, knocking *his* hat off, *her* hat askew, her long brown hair loose from its bun pinnings, and her pride down to about a minus seven on the scales of dignity. She stood, brushed herself off, straightened her hat and skirt, only to discover her knee bleeding and protruding through an enormous gaping hole in her brand new shredded pantyhose.

I picked myself up, brushed myself off and gave immediate thanks I was not wearing pantyhose and my sandal straps were intact. I repositioned a smile on my face and entered the tiny, two-chair shop. I caught my breath sharply at the expression on the face of my "Delilah," my beautician, my friend for years, Dorothy. She was smiling, too, but her eyes looked grim. I wondered if mine did. Dammit! I wish I couldn't read eyes so well. Obviously she was dreading this experience as much as I. My breathing almost stopped.

I started to chatter mindlessly, talking of anything, everything but what I was truly feeling. I even said, "Nice weather, isn't it?"—and winced inwardly. I wished I could tell Dorothy some of Michael's bull stories, but I didn't think she would appreciate them, being a very conservative, religious lady; she even had a religious tape library on the side room of her beauty shop. But every time I thought of "tastes like peppermint," I'd chuckle to myself. It kept a smile on my face.

Before the shampoo, "Delilah" struck her first scissors attack. Whack, whack—five or six inches of my hair fell to the floor—"to make it easier to shampoo," she explained matter of factly before I asked. My scalp was as numb as my mind because I didn't even feel the water at first, then it was back to the other chair for the final "parting." Shorter and shorter my tresses were cropped, and higher and higher rose my melancholy:

> *How incongruous to look much as I did ten years earlier! Eons ago it was and I've changed so much, become another creature. But now I've gone backward in time . . . Eerily I watched as I gradually began to resemble that girl of long ago. How ludicrous that a haircut could make such a difference. Dorothy seemed to me as the old silhouette artists who used to come through the neighborhood with their scissors, magically cutting black shapes into white, only now I was the living subject framed in a mirror.*
>
> *My emerging changing silhouette brought to mind the biggest change of my life, the change that came through cancer itself. I no longer have the time nor the energy to waste on negative, emotional roller coaster rides. I need energy for healing now— inside and out—not for emotional chaos, nor even for game playing.*
>
> *This confrontation with my own mortality may just be the greatest revelation of my life. Will I win? My dad called again just before I left for the haircut to tell me I will, in so many words. He always seemed to know when I was in the depths of hell itself, for it's then he'd call to talk of ordinary, positive things, to make me laugh, to let me know everything would be okay and each time we talked I felt as though I would win despite seemingly insurmountable odds.*
>
> *Despite a new kidney infection and resultant disorientation, I'm beginning to feel new stirrings of strength, feelings as gratifying as they are long-sought. It just seems like there's so little time . . .*

"All finished," Dorothy announced as she spun my chair and handed me the small mirror to survey my new/old image from all angles.

Oh, God—my newfound strength suddenly deserted me. I felt like Samson awakening—weak, stunned. It didn't *look* all that bad, but it felt dreadful. Even if it had looked terrible, it really wouldn't have mattered. It would be gone all too soon. I couldn't help but think of the irony here, of the pride all Wanslee men felt in retaining a full head of silver hair until they died, and it is the Wanslee female who will become completely bald at the age of thirty-five.

Slowly, weak-kneed, I rose from the swivel chair and stood wobbly and speechless, gazing at my shining brown-black curls being swept into a jumbled pile on the floor. I remembered my last painting session, how the brown paint spilled onto the pages, mixing with the blacks and reds. I saw my hair swirling and falling . . . and falling.

I grabbed the back of the chair to steady myself. "How much do I owe you?"

"Not a thing!" she answered cheerily. "This one's on the house."

"Thank you," I said, as I walked to the door, wondering silently if maybe she didn't expect me to survive and this was her final gesture of kindness.

I felt sick to my stomach and sat down, using the pretext of donning my blue denim cap. It was then I noticed the little dish of peppermint candies on Dorothy's desk.

"It's true what they say," I told Morris later. "A spoonful of sugar really does make the medicine go down." And strength can come from sweetness, I added to myself.

Coward that I am, I wore the denim cap for two days following.

Survival Rule #16:

Laughter is medicine. Aside from the endorphins it produces, laughter offers a surcease from the grip of pain, anxiety and fear. Indulge yourself with great doses of this wondrous elixir. If you are skeptical about laughter as painkiller and healer, read Norman Cousin's *Anatomy of an Illness* and *Head First: The Biology of Hope*. Test laughter for yourself.

XVII

RED SLEEVES

Yes, we know that when you come, we die."
                                    Chiparopai
                                    an old Yuma Indian

Images of Mangas Coloradas, "Red Sleeves," who my Dad believed to be one of the fiercest Apache chiefs, drifted through the fog in my mind. As the pink/red blood-like clouds of adriamycin swirled into the bottle of clear liquid hanging above my head, I wondered how much blood he must have spilled to earn his name. Mangas Coloradas—legend has it his very sleeves dripped blood.

My father told me that during Coloradas' reign of terror in the late 19th century, my great-grandmother, Dora Beales, crossed the desert in a prairie schooner through his territory from Colorado to central Arizona. Alone, except for two tiny children, my stout-hearted widowed great-grandmother confronted the fierceness of the Apaches, and through sheer determination and fearlessness—my dad called it "moxie"—made it safely to her destination, the White Mountains of Arizona. I can't tell you how often this heritage has given me heart, filled me with confidence. After all, her blood still coursed through my veins. I closed my eyes and tried hard to muster just a little of her grit.

The adriamycin, the blood-dripping poison that would make my hair fall out, came with the third needle. The first needle—an anti-nausea shot of Compazine—was *not* what I needed most. What I really needed was an anti-anxiety shot of anything. I'd have settled for tequila—straight. I howled with pain and outrage and cursed a time or two as the burning, stinging Compazine spread through my hip.

Morris heard me clear out in the waiting room and smiled. The bearded chemotherapist and his nurse, Sherrie, just looked wide-eyed and dumbfounded.

"I have never in all my years of medicine heard a grown woman yell like that because of a single shot." The doctor sounded genuinely amazed even through his heavy accent. Obviously he and his nurse were accustomed to "good" patients.

"I tried to warn you of my low threshold of pain," I muttered, finding it difficult not to snap.

"I believe you now, I believe you." He smiled.

The second needle hurt less but frightened me more than the first. And it took longer because the veins in the crook of my arm kept rolling, avoiding the needle. I could have sworn they were as scared as my heart. Sherrie's repeated attempts were unsuccessful. The chemotherapist finally had to insert the needle—swiftly, deftly. The tube leading from it was attached to the bottle of clear liquid slowly dripping, dripping. At first I thought my blood was turning cold from the fear of it all, but my veins were frosting from the liquid chemical ice slowly filtering through them, so freezing it felt as though my arms and especially my brain were packed in increasing layers of dry ice, and so pervasive it destroyed any vestiges of grit.

So this is what it's like to be embalmed alive, I thought as Morris came in from the waiting room to stand by my side. I tried to smile, but I was too cold, even my hands felt frostbitten. I kept looking at Morris, watching his eyes looking down at me, giving me courage from without.

Then Sherrie approached with the enormous syringe filled with adriamycin.

"That needle has to be for horses!" I grumbled, "Clydesdales most likely . . ." My blood ran colder still.

"Relax," Sherrie laughed. "I inject this into that bottle, not into you."

Easy for her to laugh, I thought. She's not the one being embalmed.

When the bottle had finally, interminably finished dripping its swirls of poison, she injected yet another syringe directly into the tube leading into my arm—this one filled with the chemicals of metheltextrate and cytoxin. After about an hour, it was over.

I didn't feel too badly when I first got up from that chair, just slightly disoriented. The Compazine caused this, they told me, and would delay the onset of the sickness for three to four hours.

Morris and I took advantage of the reprieve, and denying what was coming, stopped for pizza. What a desperately good time we had: kidding around, laughing, making "sick" jokes, we ordered sausage, mushroom and black olive pizza and I daringly ordered an icy mug of beer and took two or three long swigs. My repressors were working overtime, refusing to believe I would soon be more violently sick than I'd ever imagined anyone could possibly be—and still live. Or want to, as the saying goes.

I set my jaw when it was time to go home and walk upstairs alone to endure the unendurable. Morris looked grim. He had already suffered through four surgeries, endless weeks of radiotherapy and some of my fears. He seemed so young—too young. Although I was grateful he was by my side during the treatment, I needed to be alone to brave their brutal consequences. There would be nothing he really could do, but it was a comfort he would be close by.

Within moments after the violent retching and vomiting gripped my entire body in tremendous bed-shaking spasms, I most sincerely regretted our pizza escapade. It would be years and years before I could taste another or even smell beer without nausea rising. I hate to think what the sickness would have been like without the Matropinal suppositors I fumblingly inserted to counteract it. Crushing waves of nausea convulsed me until I vomited so continuously all I could spew was dark green bile. And still the agonizing attacks continued as though a dozen demons warred within, raging, trying to find their way out of my racked body, leaving me weak, gasping, helpless.

After several hours of this wretchedness, the demons found a new way out—severe diarrhea began. Too weak by this time to even stagger, I crawled to the bathroom dragging my "sick pan" beneath me, afraid I'd vomit enroute. I did.

As a wounded coyote drags herself through the desert back into her den to whimper and lick her wounds, waiting for healing or death, so I crawled back into my bed in a bilious, black fog, able only to slowly curl into the fetal position and tuck my sick pan under my chin.

Between onslaughts of gall, I wept helplessly and gasped and panted over and over, "Oh, God . . . oh, my God . . ." I was not crying out for mercy. I was conscious only of trying to pull Him closer to me. It was the only way I knew to avoid feeling totally abandoned by Him, as if saying his name over and over, He could not get very far from me—or forget me.

This dreary, sickening routine repeated itself again and again for the better part of three days. After the first twenty-four hour period, the violent spasms did not diminish in intensity, but gradually, ever so gradually, they lessened in frequency—until by the third day, all the horrors gave way to mere hopelessness. I just lay there befogged, prostrate and totally despairing, so racked and weakened, I had to think about it a long, long time—giving myself A, B, C directions—before I could move my arm, or more complicated yet, turn over.

All during those days, Morris quietly, tenderly checked on me, from time to time emptying the sick pan while fighting his own nausea. He bathed my face with a cool, damp cloth, and looked very sad and very lost.

And Samson, "Sam," our eight-year-old half-Beagle, half-God-knows-what-Sam, became my consistent empathetic companion. From the first hour of my sickness, he jumped up on the bed, threw himself down against me and would not leave my side. When I curled to the left or the right, he snuggled and pushed his chunky little Beagle body against my back. When I could lie flat, he'd nestle against my side and nuzzle his cold, wet nose in my armpit. When my son tried to coax him to eat or go outside, he usually refused. He'd just huddle ever closer, gazing mournfully at me, his round little body resembling a black bellows as he heaved his long, sad sighs. Sam sounded and looked as depressed as I felt. There wee moments, hours, especially when Morris was away at school, when the warmth of Sam seemed my only tangible link to the world outside my galling delirium.

Once my reformed-alcoholic father described the horrors of his own delirium tremens as he struggled to end his obsession with the evils of spirits. I listened to all his words, but understood more from the reflections in his eyes as he recounted the overwhelming despair, the nightmares, the awesome terror as torrents of sweat poured from his trembling, craving body, amid mad ravings and horrid hallucinations of giant spiders attacking him.

By the third day of my own ordeal, I felt as though I'd been through it all except for the spiders, but a creeping, mind-numbing, overwhelming depression compensated for any lack of eight-legged creatures.

By the fourth day, I could move about, albeit ever so slowly, and eat a few bites of bland foods—unbuttered toast, clear broth and plain tea. Just the thought of strong flavors of any kind, especially coffee or, oh, God! pizza and beer, triggered the nausea all over again. I was to discover that queasiness would never really leave all during the next two years—throughout intensive, intravenous chemotherapy or the year of oral treatments following.

To counteract it, I munched on nacho cheese-flavored corn chips and salted nuts. Those crunchy snacks eased the nausea and replenished the salt in my system that the chemicals destroyed. Those same salty, crunchy snacks also eased about twenty-five pounds onto my frame in less than three months, which didn't help my ongoing depression nor my shaky body image.

By the fifth day, two days before my follow-up treatment with straight injections, I knew with grave certainty it would not be chemicals that saved me. I'd be lucky if I could survive the chemicals. It would be love that pulled me through—the love of my son, my father, my brother and the love of my friends who had become mother, father, sister, brother to me. I would never be able to endure the next two and a half years of devastating, debilitating surgeries and treatments without Love beckoning me forward.

On the seventh day, as I drove our Cougar convertible through the streets of Houston to my next dreaded appointment, I seriously reconsidered my great-grandmother's courage, and wished with all my heart I were driving a prairie schooner alone through the desert to face the terrors of Mangas Coloradas.

Sharon Wanslee

Survival Rule #17:

The antidote to fear is not courage, but Love. Replace fear with
Love. Courage will naturally follow.

XVIII

AREQUIPA'S GIFT

"My greatest satisfaction from my work is to see peo-ple like you enjoying life."

Luis Televera Campos, M.D

In the land of the Inca and Machupicchu, there lies a love-ly place at the foot of the mountains in southern Peru called Arequipa. I took great courage from this place. Only one hour from the Pacific Coast, the sun shines every day all year long and the rainfall is predicted, not at nighttime as in Camelot, but between one and five o'clock every afternoon during the three months of summer. The temperature is never too cold nor too warm with only a 20 degree difference in the highs and lows, and with humidity hovering around eleven percent.

Here in this ideal place was born a physician among physi-cians—"a natural doctor" as he explains—because his father was a physician, his father's father was a physician, three of his uncles were physicians and his brother soon followed suit. It was here in Arequipa that Luis Campos came into the world— Luis Televera Campos, that intense, bearded, "Latin Peter Ustinov" chemotherapist—born amid this matrix of healers in an unequaled setting.

When he was first in Medical School, professors from Johns Hopkins University came for a year-long sabbatical in Arequipa; Campos was puzzled and asked the Chief of Cardiology, "Why?" The American doctor replied, "Arequipa is Paradise—No place in the world has this weather nor nicer people."

"Probably he was right," said Campos.

He first came to the United States in 1970 to work in the prevention of rejection of transplanted organs at UCLA. Later he formally studied internal medicine, but decided that the rejection of transplanted organs was an easy problem to conquer; he felt it would be a much greater challenge to study the rejection of tumors. This is how and why he came to M. D. Anderson Cancer Center in Houston, Texas, where he worked with Dr. Joseph Sinkovics, Oncologist/Immunologist. During the recession most grants unfortunately were lost; two years later Campos entered private practice. Dr. Sinkovics followed him in his footsteps and came to work with him.

Of course, I met Campos at Rosewood Hospital the day I learned I had to endure chemotherapy. That day I could not separate the messenger from the long-dreaded message. Knowing what he was and what he did scared me witless. And while his gravity had at first caused me terrible misgivings, it would be this same deadly serious, straight-arrow quality that gave me the most confidence for the months, the years ahead. Campos became for me a dauntless warrior against the implacable many-faced omnipresent foe called Cancer.

As he later told me, the most vital trait to become an oncologist is essentially to have the vocation, the passion for it.

"Without it," he says, "one would be a very frustrated, a very unhappy person. You have to love what you are doing and love serving people, but probably the most important aspect is that you become very close to your patients and their families.

"In my early days, I made an effort not to become engaged emotionally with my patients—to protect myself. I was wrong.

I was fighting the natural tendency to become close to them and when I realized that was what I should do, I became much happier. And I'm certain I did a better job.

"You have to be aware that you are the last stop for these patients and families and if you are not there maybe everything else is gone."

He was right. He was my last stop. Were he not there, everything else *would* be gone. And in his presence, such was his steadfast dedication and his profound compassion, he soon instilled in me the hope, the assurance that together we could and would beat back the foe.

Campos' philosophy regarding the survival of cancer patients is one of long-term goals. He feels a patient should have a realistic but optimistic position knowing that life is important and death is an irrevocable fact of life. What is most important is not necessarily when one dies, but how.

He encouraged me always to have a horizon, goals—even small goals. And he tried to discourage me from working too closely with other cancer patients until my own battle was won—realistically appraising my prognosis and balancing this with my inherent capacities for depression.

This realistic, optimistic hopeful approach translated well into my own life, maybe because it was infused with the energy radiating from the man. Once inside his office door, I never had to ask if he were in or not. I instantly knew by the energy level—or lack of it—if he were present. So catalytic is this vigorous energy, this bright stimulus, that within moments of his arrival, everyone responds with their own heightened spirit—nurses, receptionists and especially patients in the waiting room.

Burn-out doesn't set in because he copes with the on-going stresses of oncology by taking frequent breaks. A few days out of town with his family every six weeks or so seems to revitalize his energy full-strength. He returns refreshed, renewed.

Add to this on-going energy, his innovation and desire to

offer the "most up-to-date cutting-edge therapy," according to his nurses, "his highly intelligent, knowledgeable" approach, and its' easy to see how he generates confidence along with his energy.

Through it all flows that incomparable compassion for his patients that is healing in itself. We've all felt it.

One Saturday I was rushed to meet Campos in the hospital emergency room. In my zeal to combat the crushing nausea of a chemo treatment, I'd taken far too much anti-nausea medication and it severely interfered with my capacity to breathe—not a good experience if one is claustrophobic and must have an abundance of fresh air on one's face at all times.

The ER workers had just given me the injection that would stop the reaction and free my throat and lungs when Campos arrived. Only two or three minutes has passed but it seemed like forty. Still struggling for air I looked up and almost did not recognize him. Gone was the three-piece suit, replaced by jeans and guayaberas [Mexican wedding shirt]. So panicked was I by my lack of real breathing, I thought I might be hallucinating. But as the injection began to work, I could clearly see the concern in his eyes and the small cross hanging on a gold chain around his neck.

He took one of my hands in both of his and said, "You must help this shot. You must calm down so it can work. You must *do* this. *Now.*"

I was afraid to let go of his hand, so I closed my eyes and forced calm upon myself while feeling strength from him. Within moments I was serene and breathing freely.

From that point in time, I understood the determination and tenderness this physician combined to care for his patients. When I relayed this thought to him later, he grinned and said, "But that is what my initials stand for—Luis Televera Campos—L. T. C.—*"loving, tender care."*

I also understood what great good fortune I had to be in Houston, a city of international healers, where "the surgeon's surgeon," Dr. Jose Iglesias of Colombia, S. A., steered me toward Rosewood Hospital and the healing team of Drs. Vincent Patrick Collins of Toronto, Canada, and Luis Televera Campos, healing warrior and finest Peruvian gift of Arequipa.

Survival Rule #18:

Utmost confidence in your doctor is imperative. With it you can win. Without it, all the medical procedures in the world will be sabotaged by the lurking doubts in your mind. If you do not have such full trust, search until you find the physician not only worthy to be in charge of your prognosis, but of your hope as well.

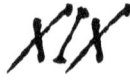

XIX

ANNA II

". . . all at once the heavy night
Fell from my eyes and I could see—
A drenched and dripping apple tree
A last long line of silver rain . . ."

"*Renascence*"

Edna St. Vincent Millay

Anna bloomed. I watched in wonder as slowly, continuously, much like a colorless chrysanthemum bud beheld through the eye of time-lapse photography, Anna unfolded petal by petal into a joyous burst of color.

After only two weeks of trial and error, Anna was truly mess painting, and she'd definitely begun confrontations with fear, anger, disappointment and sorrow. After those first two weeks, I began to wonder if this process could guide her down the road to save her own life. It would at least turn her life around. Painting strengthened her determination and resolve with a cumulative effect.

Throughout the eight weeks I guided her through the CMT course, Anna unburdened the overload of her soul. The cloudy film of ever-present tears disappeared and her eyes began to sparkle. Gradually she began to laugh—not often, but when she did it was a warm, throaty chuckle—and it was wonderful.

Anna had good reason for quiet pleasure, many good reasons: every relationship in her immediate family improved, with each of her six children and even the stormy one between her and her uncommunicative husband; she gained energy, and with it momentum for activities she'd abandoned long before; she even gained weight. For the first time in over five years, Anna tipped the scales five pounds heavier than her previous check-up.

Each day she took a long walk in the sunshine through her neighborhood, rediscovering vivid hues of flowers, foliage and sky and the quiet warmth of a neighbor's wave. When she returned home she tied with an orange ribbon around her neck a colorful green, yellow and blue placard decorated with orange tempera flowers that read: *PLEASE DO NOT DISTURB!—this is my quiet, alone time.* A houseful of eight people does not easily lend itself to silence and solitude, but the sign afforded her enough privacy from family intrusions to meditate, read, listen to music and fill her soul. The Steinway in the corner of her den, no longer silent, echoed Anna's resurgence of life for longer and longer periods each day.

Soon her house could no longer hold her and her music. She returned to church and began to play for the choir once again, not on a regular basis, but for practices, substitutions and an occasional wedding. She cooked dinner for her family now as in days of health, and her hunger for life and music sent her questing two or three afternoons a week to museums, concerts, films, or simply lunch with friends.

I had the first honor. We went to Wendy's. It was bright, informal, fast and only two blocks away. I didn't have much time. It was Anna's treat and she was craving a big, juicy, hamburger. She couldn't remember the last time she'd tasted one. Being with Anna that day was like being with a little girl discovering hamburgers, milkshakes and ordering all by herself for the first time. She even played with straws and ordered a second chocolate milkshake, all the while smiling and looking around wide-eyed, noticing everything about her new surroundings and its occupants.

I don't recall most of our exact conversation, but I do remember her smiling, sparkling eyes and the serenity that flowed from her. And the excitement. She was on her way to the Houston Museum of Fine Arts for the first time in many, many years. She'd wanted to share the trip with me, surprising me with the invitation during class that day. But I couldn't go. Within an hour I would be hooked up to my second major chemotherapy treatment—bottles, tubes, needles—with my thoughts far from Manet and his "Rainbow Bridge," or any of my other favorites Anna would be viewing.

For a moment, just a moment, Anna's eyes misted over, something I hadn't seen for a while.

"Anna, what's wrong?"

She couldn't speak for several minutes. I waited. Finally, very quietly and with great difficulty, she said, "You've given . . . me . . . so much . . ." she paused a long, long time, "understanding, friendship . . . hope . . . I mean . . . it makes me so sad . . . it's so unfair that you have to go through those . . . *treatments*." She said the word "treatments" as though she were describing a pit of rattlesnakes.

"To tell the truth, Anna, I wish I didn't have to, either. But they tell me they're necessary . . . just as I'm sure yours were." I touched her hand and tried very hard to look only at her eyes and her hands as I talked. It still struck terror in my heart to look at her hair. As short as it was, somewhere between one and two inches, it was much, much longer than mine would be for a longtime once it began to fall.

Suddenly, as if she couldn't stand this intrusion of gloom into such a happy occasion, she grabbed her purse and exclaimed "Omigosh!—I almost forgot." And with that she whipped out three Polaroid photographs and proudly handed them to me, her face beaming like a toddler home from pre-school with her crayon pictures.

I nearly lost my Wendy's hamburger and milkshake when I saw the top photo. It was a "before" shot of lesions from Anna's shingles taken some time before she began CMT—horrible, angry red encrusted, oozing blisters covering most of her right shoulder and back, and the second shot, another "before," demarcating the extensive encroachment of the same lava-like wounds under her arm and across her right breast.

The last photo, the "after" shot, revealed a proudly smiling Anna looking over her perfectly-healed shoulder and back—all smooth and healthy-looking, the scar tissue only slightly darker in pigmentation than the unaffected area.

"Each time I painted, I felt the pain easing," she told me, "until it gradually just went away."

It was my turn to get misty-eyed. In my hand I held what looked to be tangible documented proof of Anna's inner healing of mind and emotions.

As we hugged farewell until our next class meeting, Anna clung to me just for a moment. This time, however, I felt as though she were giving, not taking, courage.

Survival Rule #19:

Whine carefully. If you catalogue your woes aloud, there may be one listening who has been through much more. Or say to yourself, "That's just what they're saying in Bosnia"—or Rwanda or wherever the pocket of the world's misery happens to be at the time. This thought provides great leveling perspective to your own sufferings.

Save up real complaints to discuss with a counselor or a confidant. And choose these carefully.

XX

THE RUNNER

"A Wounded Deer—leaps highest—
I've heard the Hunter tell—
'Tis but the Ecstasy of death—
And then the Brake is still! . . . [165]

Emily Dickinson

"The Loneliness of the Long-Distance Runner"—I wonder if it begins to compare with the loneliness of the long-term cancer patient? Each face a long, long race, but for the patient there are no cheering crowds, no banners waving, only terror and misunderstanding reflected in the eyes of the spectators. No one—*not one person*—begins to understand what you are going through. Expect this, I told myself. Accept it.

"Keep a stiff upper lip." "Hang in there." "Gee, how do you take it?" "Well, now that there's no need for a biopsy, there's no need to worry, is there/" "You're handling it so well . . ." they all say at one time or another, in one way or another.

They don't realize you're running hurdles—you cleared this one, but you can see a much bigger, more formidable one ahead. And then you kick yourself for looking up the track. You get the good news on Monday that you do not need another biopsy—yet—this day, "but come back in two weeks and let's have another look."

The spectators never hear the pep rallies you give yourself, how you repeatedly tell yourself in the middle of the interminable, dark night that you've had two more biopsies since the first two terrible ones last November, and these last two proved to be negative. (Funny how if it's "negative" that's good, and if it's "positive" it's so bad as to mean sickness unto death.) But then you remember your mother's ravaged body and soul and your breathing catches again.

You wonder, alone and silently to yourself, as your chest burns each time you move, are these other lumps in your remaining breast still benign or not? Your body turns to find amore comfortable position and the bandage covering the open grid-like wound of the BCG immunology treatment you gave yourself that morning pulls and stings and hurts your hip and with each pull you're reminded of the next hurdle: another "Biggie" chemo treatment, preceded by the test hurdles— chest X-rays, EKG, innumerable blood tests and those dratted stinging, itching skin tests, needles up and down the right arm.

No one begins to suspect how you hate needles now. You used to be able to feign bravery. But chemotherapy makes the veins in your arm, your entire arm, tender and sensitive, so sensitive that the needles hurt now. A lot, dammit!—especially since the veins are now scarred. It's as if you've been scalded from the inside out. So in front of the spectators—medical people and friends—you laugh and make jokes about what a big baby you are. Meanwhile on the inside, you cringe and plead to stop the race. Your practical side counters with the quiet observance, "Thank God, they can do all these things for you." But somehow the inwardly-whining, whimpering side of you agrees, while fervently wishing everything could just stop. Now!

"They may never stop," Reality suggests. It may be one weakening race after another until Time has run out . . ." The hair that has just barely started growing back into silky peach fuzziness all over your head could disappear again if they "upped" your chemo dosage. The nodules in your right breast and axilla could prove to be more dangerous, meaning more surgery, radiotherapy and, oh, God, chemotherapy! I just don't think I could go through "The Great Fall" one more time—my hair coming out by the brushfuls and handfuls much like a woolly-dog's fur. A handful of hair left in my palm after I'd leaned my head on my hand was the first signal it was beginning. It became so much worse than I expected, so much worse than I'd been led to believe. I didn't know how to handle the cascades of falling hair. Aside from covering all my clothes, my shedding shorn locks were all throughout the sheets and pillowcases, covering the carpet, the bathroom sink and countertop, the tub and shower curtain despite all my efforts of vacuuming and cleaning. More handfuls came out as I cleaned and with each handful I wondered how much more of me the chemicals were destroying.

Surely, surely the practical and whimpering sides of you pray, you won't have to experience the Great Fall more than once, for it occurs to you that when Time has run out and only the Ultimate Hurdle remains, you would at least like to clear it with a full head of hair . . . So you keep running—from an enemy you never see. All that's visible is a body left grotesquely asymmetrical, new markings called scars, and of course, a naked scalp. You feel the terror, the pain, weakness, nausea never-ending, the isolation and the indescribable loneliness this unseen enemy causes—and you run harder.

On days when the race seems too grim, too intense and entirely uphill, I run to friends. With my dad and my brother over a thousand miles away, and my son in school, Kathleen was always the closest and most comforting to seek. Our friendship began when I taught my first CMT group class. But we became close during her mother's illness and death from pancreatic cancer. I served as Kathleen's sounding board for the frustration and grief of that painful experience, and Kathleen understood so much more of my own battle after standing by her mother through that war.

We had much in common: we were the same age, we each had worked in advertising and written for newspapers [Kathleen for the *Cleveland Plain Dealer* and *The Detroit News*], we were each at turning points in our life. She was Irish Catholic and I was Welsh-Irish and lately come, thanks to Thomas Merton and St. John of the Cross, to the Catholic faith.

But there were striking differences—from a wealthy family, Kathleen has a flair for always saying the most gracious words, While I, on the other hand, try to follow the advice of both Balzac and my father of developing one's character and then saying what you truly feel—"shooting from the hip." Unfortunately, 'what you truly feel" is often the precise something someone else may not want to hear. Perhaps my character is not prime yet. My approach to fashion usually consists of jeans, sweatshirt and sneakers—sandals in summertime— while Kathleen is simple elegance personified. And she's the truest "Superwoman" I know: married with two daughters, she juggles with ease career, homemaking, motherhood, gourmet cooking, writing and a busy social life. Yet to see her in jeans, her ash-blonde hair up in pigtails, sans makeup, sitting tailor-fashion on her sofa, sipping a glass of Bordeaux, she seems a carefree eleven-year-old.

Although it's not easy for Kathleen to share her own feelings, she is uncannily perceptive of other's moods and needs— including mine. I felt reinforced with grace and strength each time I talked with her. Lunch together once a week at Ouisie's table and The Traveling Brown Bag Lunch Company on Sunset Boulevard near Rice University became a bright warming beacon on my bleak horizon.

"How *are* you?" Kathleen would ask, her dark brown eyes searching. Such was our friendship, I felt I could level with her—except this time I didn't want to tell her all of it. My strength failing, my spirits plummeting and my hope beginning to ebb, all I managed to say was "Kathy, I'm beginning to understand the so-called "loneliness of the long-distance runner. This seems like such a long . . . lonely race . . . it seems never-ending . . .

"I know. I know . . . I don't know what my mother would have done had I not been there . . ." She looked out the window, remembering. Her eyes looked thoughtful and sad.

"Sharon, why don't you go see Ken Kopel?—that psychologist I've mentioned before. I've seen him several times for family counseling and each time I've walked away feeling so much better—better able to cope. He's young, but he's good. And I just learned he specializes in counseling cancer patients."

I dutifully wrote down his name and telephone number, promising to call him—sometime—someday—but vowing to myself I would do everything I could to handle as much as I could, as long as I could, all by myself.

"I'm sorry to complain, Kathleen. Maybe it's just that in exactly one hour and forty-five minutes I'm going to be hooked up to those dripping bottles of poison again."

"Who's going to be with you?"

"No one this time; I'm going it alone . . ." I couldn't keep myself from adding, ". . . just like the last time." I immediately winced, realizing how self-pitying that sounded.

"No!" She shook her head. "Oh, no, you're not! I'm going with you."

"But, Kathleen . . ."

"I'll simply call my office," she said. And she simply did.

She stood beside me all during that treatment, imparting strength and caring, the gift of her presence. In one afternoon, Kathleen taught me that the single most important act a friend can offer a cancer patient is to *be there*. Words are not necessary nor are gifts. Even cards with notes of encouragement pale beside the simple, courageous act of being present during another's loneliness, fear and pain. From that moment, between my son and Kathleen, I never again faced the increasingly frightening chemotherapy sessions alone. So much for my plaint of "not one person" understanding.

Unfortunately, nothing cold allay my fears of the black, bilious mini-death that followed, leaving me weaker each time. To counteract it, to feel more alive, to feel more in control when it was over, I tried literally to become a long distance runner. I started a jogging program, actually a walking program with a few jogging steps thrown in. Brand new tan and white Nike running shoes helped inspire me.

O Nike, Goddess of Victory, help me be victorious in this race I'm running.

At first I managed to jog only seven steps—I counted them because each stride took such forceful effort. After seven, my knees, my legs and my head felt so wobbly I could hardly stand, much less walk, and hard as I tried, I couldn't keep from loudly gasping for air as I doubled over, holding onto my knees for support. But I did manage to keep my wig in place with a blue kerchief tied peasant style around my "hair." It didn't feel good wearing it while getting hot and sweaty, in fact it itched horribly against my bare scalp, but I was convinced it made me *look* "normal and healthy." that had become so important to me. God, how I wanted to be normal and healthy!

Each day I determined to add seven more steps until I could jog at least a whole block at a time. What exhilaration when I succeeded! I kept pushing my distance, my stamina in the months that followed as I jogged through the streets of West University. Roses and puppies always caught my eye along the way. They heartened me by just "Being"—living reminders of the beauty and spontaneous joy of life in spite of it all. They gave me an extra burst of energy and just for a moment or two I would really fly. Hope is anywhere you can find it.

With each succeeding month, I kept pushing back the goal, jogging two or three miles at a stretch. I actually felt I was beginning to outdistance my invisible enemy.

And each day as I started down the block, I'd remember what Jesse Owens said about running. I'd interviewed him once for an article for *Up With People News* (he served as board member); and I asked him if he said any particular prayer to help him run, particularly when he ran in the 1936 Olympics before his foe of all foes—Adolf Hitler, who wanted this Black man defeated at all costs. Owens smiled and answered, "Yes, just one—'Lord, if you'll keep pickin' 'em up, I'll keep layin' 'em back down.'"

Survival Rule #20:

Progress will be indicated by a zigzag line not a straight one. A few days of confidence and vitality may be followed by days of depression and total prostration. That's okay. It's all part of the healing process.

Never, NEVER assess your life, your situation, your medical prognosis at night. If you are already experiencing the dark night of your soul, don't plunge yourself deeper into the shadows. Too many fears are born in the gloom of exhaustion and discouragement.

Fill your evening and night hours with as much comfort, joy, love, laughter, rest and renewal as possible. Your body needs this time for healing purposes. Your mind and your soul need to be replenished by courage, goodness and peace.

Reserve time early in the morning every day to worry. Set an alarm for a half-hour. Write down each and every worry or dire thought you can imagine. When the alarm rings, slam the notebook shut. Put it and your fears away for another twenty-four hours. When your cancer challenge is over, you will be amazed at how few of those anxieties materialized.

XXI

TRUE FRIEND

A faithful friend is a sure shelter,
whoever finds one has found a rare treasure.

Ecclesiastics 6:14

Jerusalem Bible

I couldn't run long enough, far enough, fast enough. After a few months yet another biopsy caught up with me.

Whom do I tell? To whom do I run and complain this time? With which of my loved ones, my friends, my acquaintances do I share this new terror? Certainly not Morris—he needs positive news now; not my family in Arizona, meaning my brother and father— they would only panic, drop everything and rush to Houston, where there would be absolutely nothing they could do. Not friends. How long can you go on chronicling the unraveling of a body, of a life, before they say, "I just can't take anymore." I thought about Kathleen's suggestion: I found the address and number and called Ken Kopel, her psychologist friend, and made an appointment for the following Wednesday evening.

When I entered Kopel's office in a highrise on Hillcroft at 7:30, I was dismayed to see a small handwritten note taped to the receptionist's window. It read—*Dr. Kopel is running a little late.*

"Well, just well!" I said to myself.

I sat in a leather chair, looked at all the abstract art on the walls and perused his magazines, all current and up-to-date.

More time passed, about forty-five minutes. I worked a crossword puzzle in the *Houston Post* and seriously considered bolting at least three times. I don't need this, I thought, as I picked up my purse and nearly made a clean get-away, when the inner door finally opened.

A young well-dressed man appeared and aid my name as a question. He looked much more youthful than I imagined and in retrospect I can only describe him as a young Tom Hanks-type: spare of frame, curly light brown hair and big blue eyes that seemed intense, inquisitive and kind.

"Please, go in and have a seat. I'll be right with you."

Okay, okay, I thought, as I sat down in his inner office facing a west window and a burgeoning red hibiscus plant. I'll see it through one session. After that I'll play it as a variation of Pasal's Wager: Live life as though God exists, said Blaise Pasal, the 17th Century philosopher. If you reach the end of your life and discover there really is, you will have gained Eternity. Conversely, if you reach the end of your days and find there is no God, you will have lost nothing, but you will have lived a more altruistic and fulfilling life. In this counseling milieu, I would trust that Dr. Kopel would offer insight and solace to me. If he could, I will have gained strength, and perhaps, even courage to live or die. If not, I will have lost nothing, but perhaps gained some understanding along the way.

"Tell me why you're here," he began.

"My friend Kathleen told me that you specialize in counseling cancer patients."

"That's one of my specialty areas in behavioral medicine—along with cardiac, dialysis and other medical patients."

I catalogued my medical situation, all the surgeries and chemotherapy treatments, along with the stresses of divorce, that were gradually grinding me down into a creature of no energy, no joy, no hope—no hair.

He looked at my "hair," and said. "A wig?"

I nodded, and his expression softened from professional interest to understanding compassion.

"To tell you the truth, Doctor, (it seemed strange to call someone so young "doctor") I feel like jumping off a porch."

He looked at me quizzically.

"Well, I don't quite feel desperate enough to jump off a cliff. I may want to think things over. So I believe I'd like to jump off a real high porch."

We laughed together. I liked him. And by the end of that first session, I knew I'd found a friend. Before long, I would discover that, although he may have looked like a young Tom Hanks, he proved to be as compassionate and wise as a mature King Solomon. He was a born psychologist—brilliant, intuitive and infinitely compassionate. And very funny. Like Campos, he knew as early as the eighth grade what his vocation would be, when he chose "psychologist" on "career day."

When I asked him if he followed any particular school of thought in his work, he smiled and told me, "I'll use any and all schools—including the kitchen sink—if I think it will work."

From that first day forward, I found this to be true. Using all his psychological skills from all the schools, he could read me like a familiar manuscript. He guided me, challenged me, heartened me, consoled me, encouraged me—and through it all he not only helped me cope, he helped my spirit grow. He followed me through all the medical crises and laughed and cried with me when I conquered them.

I tried to see him before each chemotherapy treatment, and each time he fortified me for the ordeal. When yet another biopsy crisis seemed too formidable, he told me to seek the book, *Hope for the Flowers*, by Trina Paulus, a children's book written for adults all about caterpillars finding courage enough to become butterflies, about willingness to lose everything by entering a chrysalis and trusting. It not only worked, I've given away dozens of copies of *Hope* through the years.

This young psychologist reminded me that you cannot wait for joy until life gets better. You have to find or make joy while in the midst of sorrow, fear, even depression. "Go to the zoo," he told me. "Buy a bunch of balloons, watch all the animals, let the balloons go one by one or all at once and feel their freedom.

"Build a support system of both female and male friends. Tell them what you're doing and why you chose them. Buy a poster that makes you feel good, that reminds you of joy, and put it up in an unlikely place where you'll see it many times a day.

"Take at least thirty minutes a day, an hour is better, to do nothing but that which pleases you. And stop isolating yourself—go to movies, go to plays, concerts. Plan outings with friends. Stop postponing living."

I did it all—the list of friends, the plays, the movies, the zoo with its graceful giraffes, mating hippos, obscene monkeys and balloons that I freed to the sky one by one to prolong the exultant feeling. I bought a new suit and a new poster of a soaring rainbow-hued hot air balloon entitled, "Freedom."

I started living again. I stopped defining myself by a disease. Instead, joy slowly filtered back into my life. I even began buying flowers, inspired no doubt by the ever-present red hibiscus plant blooming in Kopel's window.

How bizarre it seems to me that a person, particularly one in public life, is considered suspect if they've had psychological counseling. Wouldn't it make more sense to applaud them for mending a broken part of their life? Wouldn't it make more sense to consider suspect anyone who does *not* seek counseling—we are all broken somewhere, some way. How much less evil would we experience? How much safer would our society be if we all led *examined* lives? All it took for me to appreciate this was to find what lay hidden deep in my own heart of darkness, unknowing, until Wolfgang Luthe and Ken Kopel guided me into their lights of seeing and understanding.

What a paradox—we'll pay enormous sums of money to experts who advise us about computers, cars, investments and even clothes, yet concerning our children, our marriages, our minds, our very souls, we figure we'll just wing it.

With enormous medical bills that climbed weekly and no insurance, thanks to a divorce, I'd soon be winging it myself. No money was left for counseling. I told Kopel.

"Don't worry about it. We'll take care of it later," was all he said. "Later" proved to be a couple of years down the road—I paid as much of the bill as I could then, and Kopel wrote off the rest. He wanted to see me through the on-going crisis. And so he did.

Over the years, I've sent many other people to see him, and when I feel there's too much stress in life and I need a good sounding board, I return to that fifth story office with its red hibiscus blooming. From that same west window I've attached countless beautiful sunsets—one of Kopel's favorite things in life, sunsets. They're not as fiery here as they are in my native desert, but I think for him they are a symbol of completion.

From time to time I'm amused to see that same "late" message at the receptionist's counter, but it's now a typeset plaque, matted and framed: "Dr. Kopel is running a little late, so please make yourself comfortable." For me it's a symbol of his dedication. He never stops in the middle—if your problem is too complex, he'll see it through with you.

There's a maturing silver at his temples now, but he still looks like a young Tom Hanks. He became for me a friend for life. And Kathleen was right. I never set foot into Ken Kopel's office without feeling a whole lot better about living *and* dying when I walked out, and the wisdom he gave me proved to be one of the surprising, saving graces of my life.

Survival Rule #21:

Find a counselor worthy to be called True Friend. And if you can, see your counselor before any major treatment or medical procedure. This fortification will surprise you with its strength.

Then find a new notebook and reserve it for all those thoughts that are life-giving and filled with hope, for all those ideas that come to you while reaching out to Life, for funny sayings, cartoons or happenings, or for inspiring ones. Refer to it often. Call it your "Survival Journal."

XXII

MORRIS COOL

My son, be attentive to my words;
incline your ear to my sayings . . .
Let your eyes look directly forward,
and your gaze be straight before you.

Proverbs 4:20 & 25

Oxford Annotated Bible

How I missed the "Professeur." I wanted to see his eyes shining when I told him about Anna and her progress. How I loved to bring to light Luthe's gentle, tender side. Not many people se it. They only see his implacable dedication to strip reality to its barest bones. An unpopular job at best, it's one that requires great inner strength. He has it, of course. *Do I?*— I asked my journal. *Is my inner strength sufficient to withstand the "dirty tricks" of all the people I'm teaching? I'll find out soon enough.*

My first group class of eight people began in mid-April. Seven were chosen by Fr. Monahan, from his self-actualizing "Omega Seminar," as the most receptive, the most open to new paths.

Kathleen was the eighth. She'd never taken an Omega course, yet she became the most promising student, making the first painting breakthrough. Her enthusiasm was closely followed by Frank, who had reason to be hopeful about the course. He had leukemia and less than five years to live, or so the doctors told him. Three others seemed eager, two appeared to be slightly skeptical and one wary, if not downright hostile.

No one had a thing to lose except time, which Frank was hoping to gain. Their course fee would be refunded at the end of the six weeks, a move the good Father deemed necessary for this prototype class, a necessary incentive to complete the course. In reviewing the explicit instructions with them, I made a mental note to begin my own disciplined painting schedule. Lately, I'd only sporadically thrown paints, while studying and trying to prepare a work manual I'd discussed with Luthe.

How I wished he were there to guide me. But guidance had to come from somewhere inside—that would befit Luthe's definition of creativity.

> *Soon, I vowed to my journal, soon, God willing. I want to be completely self-sufficient, able to survive and make my way without asking a single individual for help—for ANYTHING—but it's going to take a lot of work.*
>
> *There's a Ft. Apache saying for this: 'Learn to take care of yourself,' my father always told me, 'and you'll do the world a hell of a favor' . . .*
>
> *But the favor may be a bit delayed. This chemotherapy trek continues to wind ever backward and downward on the energy scale. I take one step forward, it knocks me two steps back. Some days I take one step, and it knocks me back three or four. Sometimes it's no steps forward at all. Just losing ground—falling, stumbling . . .*

A wonderful respite from such seriousness was teaching Morris to parallel park. Never was there such an eager pupil— a big, happy sixteen-year-old pup behind the wheel of our five-year-old Cougar convertible.

The quiet tree-lined streets of our West University neighborhood became his Mesa training grounds. Morris had always gotten a big kick out of my capacity to outstrip most men we knew in parallel parking—one poor fellow used to slam the car door in disgust after several futile tries and watch from the sidewalk as I neatly, effortlessly, lined p the car for him. And ever since Morris started taking driver's training at LaMar High School, he'd become even more impressed with my talent for parking. Even in the tightest spaces and the heaviest traffic, only two turns of the steering wheel, one smooth motion whipped the car into perfect position about six inches from the curb.

"Even my driving instructor can't do that, Mom. How do you do it?"

"I had a good teacher." And I explained that maybe it was because his parking lesson was there among those cool, quiet boulevards, paved streets with curbs for the eye to gauge distance, in our hold—*but still good*—Cougar convertible with automatic transmission. Whereas my parking lesson was in a four-wheel-drive ex-army jeep with a very stiff clutch out in the middle of the hot Aura Valley desert west of Tucson—way south of Old Tucson and "High Chaparral" country.

"Here you and I have other cars to judge timing and distance. Way back then, 'the olden days' as you like to call them, my instructor set up an old rusted barrel to use as the left-rear fender of the front car."

"What'd he use for the back car?"

"Your grandfather—*he* was my instructor and *he* was the left front fender of the back car. He just stood there. He never flinched—not even when that stubborn old clutch slipped several times making the jeep lurch. He stood his ground, all the while talking quietly, confidently to me, encouraging me much the way he'd talk if he were gentling a horse.

"I was scared. One false start and I knew I'd run right over him. But his trust that I could do it was infectious. After three or four tries, I believed I could do it. And I did. Your grandfather just grinned, tipped back his ever-present Stetson, looked around at the hills, distant mountains, sagebrush and sky and puffed on his cigar, while I continued to practice—at first sweating bullets and then, getting the hang of it, and feeling so happy not only because of my accomplishment, but because he looked so proud. The secret's really all in the timing . . .

"In retrospect, the only indication that your grandfather may not have been as cool as he wanted me to believe was the presence of his rope. Most of it was coiled over his left shoulder while he threw a lasso over any and all possible targets, easily, almost lazily, as if his mind were many miles or many years away. His lack of concern was inspiring."

Morris learned rapidly. I don't know if he was such a great pupil or I was such a good instructor. I didn't have a rope or a cigar, but it probably helped that I'd painted away any tensions before his lesson. My nerves were as steady as the concrete curbs he kept bumping, scraping and defacing with black tire marks.

When the lesson was complete and Morris had joined the illustrious ranks of perfect parallel parkers, he was ravenous, as only a teenager can be. Down came the top of the Cougar, unveiling the vivid blue Texas sky viewed through the interlacing oak branches overhead. What a welcoming vista to eyes weary of bumpers and fenders as he wheeled through the streets of West University and River Oaks near his school.

My long, rainbow-colored silk scarf kept my hair in place—that is, it firmly anchored my wig—and as the scarf ends fluttered in the wind I felt a little like Aurora Greenway, Larry McMurtry's unforgettable matron from "Terms of Endearment." The main difference, of course, being that in this case, the mother has the killer disease, not the child. And for this, Dear God, I am most decidedly grateful.

Morris was famished, but Morris was cool. As he wheeled

into the Jack-in-the-Box on Kirby Drive, I suddenly realized this was his first time to order fast food from the driver's seat. His voice deepened, suddenly mellowed and matured before my very ears, as he told the clown in the speaker he wanted two cheeseburgers, a large strawberry milkshake, a large order of fries and two apple pies. I ordered iced tea. As we drove up to the window, Morris spotted several of his school chums sitting at the sidewalk tables in front of the restaurant—boys and girls, about a half-dozen of them.

"Hey, Morris! How's it goin'?" "Hi, Morrie . . ."

My son grinned and waved in a new, nonchalant, off-hand style that reminded me of his grandfather and gave the clerk at the window several dollars and drove past his friends—waving, smiling, swashbuckling—out into the traffic on Kirby Drive.

"That was impressive, Morris. You handled that well."

"Mom?"

"Yes?"

"Mom, I forgot the food!"

"I know."

"Mom, I can't go back! I'm too embarrassed!"

"I know, son. Don't look back. Just keep movin' on."

Survival Rule #22:

"Stop postponing living."

Live fully in The Now. *This moment is all there is.* Live it wholly, heart, mind and soul.

XXIII

ARMEN

I am not resigned to the shutting away of loving
hearts in the
*   hard ground*
So it is, and so it will be, for so it has been, time out
of mind . . .

"Dirge Without Music"
Edna St. Vincent Millay

Sometimes the greatest gift to another is to do nothing—a lesson I learned from Armen [pronounced *ar-MAHN*].

He walked slowly into Rosewood's radiotherapy clinic. He seemed hesitant and fearful. Tall, slender with a noble face and dark, wavy hair, he would have looked much like an Arabian prince, if he hadn't seemed so scared. He looked as terrified as I felt the first time I walked through those doors.

He was alone. It was late afternoon. We were the last two patients of the day. He sat down across the room from me on the edge of the chair, his hands braced on his knees, looking straight ahead. I couldn't bear his fear. I crossed the room and sat down beside him.

"Don't be scared," I said, reaching down to touch his hand. "There's nothing to be afraid of."

His smile began slowly—trusting—lighting his eyes.

We became friends, kindred spirits. He had a young wife, two small children and cancer of the stomach. It was bad. We would see each other often at Rosewood as our treatments coincided. We would pour out our worst fears to one another in the waiting room. He was afraid he would not be able to withstand the sickness from the treatments, and I was afraid I could not withstand seeing, without identifying too strongly, the worst stages of debilitation of the other patients. I tried to give him courage and he tried to lighten my spirit. And then for a long time I didn't see him. The last time ever I saw Armen he gave me one of the finest gifts I've ever received. Late that night I wrote about it:

"Armen, In Life"

Armen, in Life
How beautiful your eyes
Enormous and brown and sensitive and kind
and so filled with fear the first time we talked.
'Don't be scared,' I said to you that first day.
'There's nothing to be afraid of,' as I touched your hand
Silently praying that this could be true for you.

Armen, in Life
How wonderful your smile
spreading slowly from your generous mouth
to your sad brown eyes
Lightening, brightening them with momentary peace.
You believed me—in the beginning.

Armen, in Life
You taught me courage
You were the one who faced the savage suffering,
All the pain,
All that wasting away
with quiet dignity and bravery and great Grace.

All reflected in your incomparable brown eyes
painfully knowing pain
yet deep and serene.

Armen, in Life,
Near the end,
Your eyes were all I recognized.
How gaunt your face—
with its hollow, hollow cheekbones.
How wasted your body—
Your clothes hanging in folds and gathers
from your slight and bending frame.

Armen, in Life,
Near the end,
I thought you were a stranger,
an old and beaten and dying man
sitting across from me in the waiting room—
Your hair just beginning to grow back
after your terrible bouts with retching chemotherapy,
Your beard—bravely cultivated
to offset the horrible physical ravaging—
heavily streaked with gray.

Armen, in cowardice,
I tried not to notice you.
I felt your pain too strongly.
Reality came roaring in on a rampage again,
And I, one of the lucky ones,
Who usually tried to smile and talk
and encourage the others,
Sat in stunned silence,
My eyes staring blindly at the pages of my book,
Trying desperately not to see
This spectre of death

Sharon Wanslee

Sitting across from me . . .
This old and beaten and dying man.
I was wrong about everything except the dying.

They called your name.
You rose painfully from your chair—
You looked at me
with your still beautiful brown eyes.
The shock of recognitions truck—
Stunned me—
Pierced me—
Armen!
Not old and beaten,
but yes, dying.

You knew who I was.
You knew, yet remained silent.
Your one quick tentative glance said it all—
You knew what it could do
were I to know it was you.
And you chose to remain alone in silence
rather than impart any suffering—
even though to share it
would diminish it . . . momentarily.
I ran after you.

Armen, in the Sunshine,
I'm so grateful to God,
We had those few moments,
Laughing and sharing our fears and our pain,
but mostly our hope.
I'm infinitely grateful God gave me
the courage to follow you—
to grasp your hand

and ask how your spirits were—
to reach out and playfully brush my hand across
your new baby-fine hair.
Mine was only a little longer then.

We left smiling—
going our separate ways.
Your eyes pleading silently,
'Be brave—
despite what you see . . .'
My heart praying, beyond hope,
that you could be spared.
I have looked for you
and prayed for you
ever since.

Armen, in death,
You are far from us now—
But peaceful, unafraid, unsuffering,
and, I like to think, smiling once again—
And I, in Life, am
Grieving.
No longer can I see
Your soul shining through
Your warm brown eyes.
Your lovely, lingering smile
lingers only in mind.

Yet the Beauty and the Courage
Your Soul brought so briefly to mine
I will try to keep shining
Forevermore,
Armen, in Life.

Survival Rule #23:

The ultimate healing is death. Make peace with this reality and with the thought that none of us gets "outta this alive."

But remember, as the body dies, the spirit grows. And so does Love. Love transcends Death.

XXIV

DREAMSCAPE

"Yet if Hope had flown away
In a night or in a day
In a vision, or in none,
Is it therefore the less gone?"
"A Dream Within A Dream"
Edgar Allen Poe

"I woke to black flak and the nightmare fighters . . ."
"The Death of the Ball Turret Gunner"
Randall Jarrell

What a horrible dream . . . My heart pounded still and I caught my breath in scary gulps. My gown and pillow and bald head were drenched in sweat . . .

Somehow in this dreamscape there was an achievement hierarchy in life, a system that acknowledged those who strived and overcame obstacles—who achieved perfection. Those who performed without stinting, without hesitation or failure were rewarded with promotion to the next level of Being, a place of increasing Peace, Wisdom, Joy and of course, great Love. Those who failed, who slipped just one time, were demoted to the next lowest level of this transcendence stratosphere.

In this dream—this nightmare—my efforts had been such,

I approached the ultimate level of this strange state of Being, and with superhuman effort of will I catapulted myself to the highest pinnacle. I looked around with great relief and joy, grateful to have reached this point where I found no sickness, no pain, no sorrow—just Love. Bliss. I could see forever.

But I slipped and fell. And the cruelest part of this surrealistic drama was its merciless price for falling from the point most sublime—one fell back not just one level, but to the base—to be broken completely—to start the long, arduous climb all over again. As I tumbled down my body broke, but as I landed at the very bottom, it was my spirit that most painfully shattered. How does Sisyphus bear it without Hope? I don't care what Camus wrote—I *cannot* "imagine Sisyphus happy."

I awoke—panting—vividly recalling the images. It was only a nightmare . . . just a dram . . . Thank God . . . Oh, thank You God . . .

Oh, God!—it's not a dream . . . Even with my eyes wide open, the nightmare continued . . . with even more intensity. Tests yesterday morning at Rosewood revealed that the dark seepage from my right breast is black blood. Many more tests revealed this nodule to be cancer. More cancer. And that means another mastectomy, more radiotherapy and two more years of chemotherapy.

I was almost There. I had almost made it. It took two and a half years for twenty-two rounds of chemotherapy. Sometimes weeks, a month, were skipped because my white blood count was too low or I was too sick and weak. I finally pleaded with Campos to stop the treatments.

His eyes compassionate, he asked, "How many have you had now?" He started checking my voluminous charts.

"Twenty-one." I didn't need a chart. "Please stop—they're killing me . . ."

He studied the chart for a long time. "It's a fine line we walk—how do you call them, those people who balance on a rope?"

"Tightrope walkers?"

"That's right, tightrope walkers. That's what we are. How much of this treatment we give you before it starts killing too many of the healthy cells? It's very difficult this walk, and sometimes our best guide is the patient. When you tell me 'it is killing me.'"

He studied the chart a while longer.

"I will make a deal with you. You take this treatment—here, today. And it is the last one."

"Thank you." I reached out and hugged him close.

I took it. I endured it. I thought I had made it. Now this. Now!—*just two weeks later*. My dream, the heartbreaking nightmare was true.

As I drove away from the clinic, I'm sure I must have looked as defeated as Anna the first time I saw her. I certainly felt that broken.

I drove North out of the city. I wanted to see Salvatore. I knew I had to drive more carefully than usual—hadn't I always told my students that a mind overburdened with stress is like a drunk on the highway? I drove more slowly, more defensively than I ever had. I was courteous—overly polite. I was even overly polite to the drunken driver of that van that broadsided me on FM 1960, a van filled with drunken hippies and illegal aliens—they must have been illegal for they careened out of that van and flew to all corners of the wind like so many bees from a fallen hive. The scene reeked of beer.

My car wasn't totaled, but it was undrivable—and so was I. Needless to say, I never saw Salvatore that day. I was grateful just to see the police and the tow truck arrive.

"I never even saw them coming," I told the officer. "Two lanes of traffic had stopped, waiting for the light and making room for me to make a left hand turn into Jim's restaurant. Too late—it was too late—by the time I saw them coming straight at me. I *thought* those truck drivers were a bit overly enthusiastic waving at me. They were trying to warn me about those drunken lunatics . . .

I never saw this new cancer nightmare coming either. Broadsided by something I can't even see . . .

Survival Rule #24:

Setbacks, even devastating ones, are inevitable in the painfully slow progress toward Victory. Don't anticipate them, but don't be thrown by them either. There will be a solution. Help will be found. Keep your eyes not on the setback, only on the prize of Victory.

XXV

FLIGHT

"I fled Him, down the nights and down the days;
I fled Him, down the arches of the years;
I fled Him, down the labyrinthine ways
Of my own mind; and in the mist of tears
I hid from Him . . ."

"The Hound of Heaven"

Francis Thompson

I ran away. Not for keeps. Just for a while. A friend loaned me his car and I fled to Corpus Christi—to Padre Island.

Space and time and silence were what I needed to cure this shock. To be alone. To sort through things. What a weak word—"things"—used for life and death and cancer and disfigurement and sickness and sorrow.

The drive didn't seem tiring until I reached Refugio, but by the time I reached Corpus Christi, exhaustion overwhelmed me. I didn't even make it to the beach. I barely made it to the bed to crash. The next day would be time enough to sit by the sea. For someone who never even saw the ocean till the age of 14, it's a rare privilege to experience that infinite expanse and watch the surf pounding in to shore. And in every direction I looked I saw scores and scores of seagulls—swooping, soaring, diving, clamoring for food, for life.

Lost in thought, in memories, mainly fearful ones, I didn't
see the young man approach, so it startled me when he spoke.

"Whenever I watch ocean waves," he said quietly, standing
just to the right and behind me, "I think of love." Annoyed
that someone would intrude upon my silence, I glanced back
at him, an average-looking guy, with an average build, light
brown hair, wire-rim glasses—and of course, I thought, oh,
swell, here's a novel approach. I hoped he would just go away.

After a moment he said, "Man loves as a trickling stream
of water. But God loves like what you see out there—with an
immensity, a power and a depth that is immeasurable, ever-
returning, eternal. Can you sense it?"

I never said a word. Chill washed over me as I watched and
heard and felt that thunderous, never-ending love of God—
mesmerized by its infinite rhythm. With every resounding
breaker that hurled itself to the beach,—rumbling, reverting
and exploding in a crescendo of white foam and spray, inun-
dating, changing all in its path, I felt more and more at peace.
An ever deepening realization of the incomprehensibility and
power of God's love engulfed me. I lost track of time. When I
looked back, the sun was setting behind towering thunder-
heads silhouetted in gold. The young man was gone.

That gift of profound peace ameliorated the shock, softened this latest blow and stayed with me until I drove back
through Houston late the following afternoon. However, the
frenetic pace of city traffic made me jumpy all over again, especially when someone edged too close to the right side of the
car. And when I drove past FM 1960, the road where the acci-
dent and my first four surgeries took place and the next one
was planned, fear slowly began to grip my heart and mind with
its freezing, relentless grip. By the time I arrived back home
that night, my weariness resulted as much from battling mental stupor and wrestling the dark angel of fear as it did from
fighting traffic. My fear was such that I felt there would be no
remedy, no hope until the surgery was over. If then.

But my greatest disappointment lay in not being able to guard the peace, the deep solace I'd found in Corpus Christi. By then the next morning I placed a call to Salvatore.

Survival Rule #25:

Run away—for a little while. If pressures grow too great, if too much advice and too many decisions overwhelm you, and you are too depleted physically and emotionally to make sense of any of it, maybe you need to run away and find your own Corpus Christi.

Simply escape. Find time for peace and solitude. Then simply return prepared for another round of the cycle of healing.

XXVI

SALVATORE

"Lord, make me an instrument of your peace . . ."
St. Francis of Assisi

Father Salvatore de George reminds me of St. Francis, primarily because of his gentleness and his willingness to cut through superficiality with bare-bones truth. He even looks a little like images of the fifteenth century Italian saint with his swarthy good looks, his intent dark-eyed gaze and his dark hair bristled around his head like a dark halo sprinkled with light.

At the Desert House of Prayer in the Tucson Mountains, a mosaic icon of St. Francis hangs on the south wall of the chapel; it looks to me like a portrait of Salvatore. But unlike a motionless icon on a wall, this Italian priest, an Oblate [Gift] of Mary Immaculate, displays incredible non-stop energy. No matter the project, for the church or for his flock, Salvatore never allows progress to bog down in committee. He simply says, "Let's do it!" and it gets done.

Despite his industry during the too-short-time he was our pastor, he always found time for personal, quiet moments, to talk to us, hug us, dipping his head down and placing it against our own in that unique way of his. And he always fed the birds.

Fr. de George—di Giorgio in the old country— is deeply

spiritual, with an attitude. His is a reverent spirituality that is as pragmatic and no-nonsense as it is somewhat skeptical of people's motives or false piety. Maybe it's because he's heard too much in too many confessionals to be otherwise.

I've always felt there's something symbolic in the way Salvatore never "preaches" from the pulpit, but simply talks to us as he steps down from the altar to our level to begin. Some of the best and most surprising homilies I've heard come from his mass celebrations. It's uncanny how he can talk on a comprehensive level to all those in his parish as disparate as many intellectual university professors, (and a few who profess to be) and the barely literate who never made it as students, and very young children, whom he always invites to sit around the altar steps as he begins his "conversation." He has a great talent to tell a story about something he recently experienced, and how it always reminds him of what Jesus meant when he said, "Love one another," or "Be not afraid," or "Seek and you shall find." His correlation of the Biblical then and the prosaic now seems masterful. And it is always surprising. Somehow I am always caught off guard. He just sounds like the same friend who talks while we gather round on kitchen stools in his rectory—making us laugh, moving us, teaching us. Only when he turns to climb the altar steps to begin the most sacred part of the mass do I realize—"He did it again—that was another homily."

My favorite recollection of this priest friend occurred one rainy Saturday morning when I accidentally stumbled into an acolyte initiation program in the sanctuary of St. Thomas. The front third of the church was filled with mothers and their youngsters—exasperated and rambunctious respectively. Had they only been speaking different languages it might have been a modern depiction of the Tower of Babel. Since they weren't, it was merely bedlam. And through all the noise, laughter, spit wads and games of tag over the pew tops, Salvatore managed to convey the necessary beginning instructions. Finally, after countless interruptions, a frazzled priest dismissed his little angels. As they burst out the side door of the church, Salvatore heaved a great sigh upon the altar, clasped both hands to his chest in a prayerful stance, lifted his eyes heavenward to the seven-foot crucifix at a compassionate Jesus looking down at him and fervently, joyfully exclaimed, "Thank You, Jesus, that I am celibate!"

His caring and gentleness belie his intensity and his cutting sense of humor. And to offset the grimness sometimes presented by the life-and-death struggles of his flock, he takes refuge in his faith, of course, but also in poets, especially Irish poets, and in music—classical music, Irish folk ballads, and artists as diverse as Joan Baez and Luciano Pavorotti.

While waiting for Salvatore that morning I put Pavorotti on the stereo, listening twice to "Nessun Dorma" and the lyrics "Al alba, vencero"—"At dawn, I will conquer . . ." Only words, I thought. Just empty, mocking words. They usually moved me to tears, but now . . .

"I'll be right there," Salvatore said on the phone. And although it was just a few minutes, it seemed at least half a day before I heard his knock.

He was very quiet as he walked in. I made tea. I needed a simple ordinary task to buffer me from the realities of more disfigurement and possible death from treatments that, despite all the sickness they induced, did *not* seem to work.

"What is it that frightens you the most about all this?" he asked.

I didn't have to search for an answer. "I'm terrified of ending up like my mother," I told him. "All that surgery, all the body parts taken—and the final coma . . ."

"Tell me about that . . . What is the scariest thing about a coma?"

At first I looked at him as though he were mad. What *isn't* scary about a coma?—I thought. But when I realized he really wanted a serious answer, I covered my eyes with my hands and tried to envision what it would be like . . . the stillness, the black nothingness, not even the beingness of a coma—"Oh, God!" I blurted out. "I never realized it before this moment, but I feel as though it's—it's just taken me so long to feel close to God—like when I used to call out 'God—O my God!' through all my chemotherapy treatments. I wasn't calling for help, Salvatore. I just didn't want to lose sight of Him, you *know?* I wanted to be *aware* of that great spiritual connection at every moment."

"And . . .?"

"And, don't you see?—if I were to fall into a coma, I could no longer be aware of Him, I'd be so lost, because I'd lose sight of Him!"

Salvatore set down his cup.

"Sharon," he paused a moment or two, "do you think God would lose sight of *you* then?"

I just looked at him. I didn't say a word. But in that silence I felt waves of serenity begin to wash over me from the top of my head down through my neck and shoulders and solar plexus down my back all the way to my toes until all the anxiety-tied knots in my skull and body unwound and flowed freely into an incredible peace. My scrunched up facial muscles relaxed and my stomach stopped hurting. It was as though I were back on the beach at Corpus Christi watching, feeling the tide and breakers wash over me.

I started to laugh. It suddenly seemed so ludicrous. Why didn't *I* think of that? Years of anguish might have been spared me. I knew that this thought was not the whole answer to my fear, yet Salvatore's simple—nearly simplistic—question began to thaw my near-frozen heart.

Do I think God loses sight of me then? No. Not now. Not even in a coma. Not ever.

Salvatore had done it again, delivered another of his incomparable homilies, but this time with only a single line. Without actually reciting scripture, Salvatore conveyed to me the assurance that I was as looked after as the least of any raven or lily-of-the-field. And I somehow knew that not only was I as cherished as any fallen sparrow, but every hard-won hair on my head was counted. I let go. I let go. *I just let go.* I released all my anxieties, all the fears that had frozen me fast for days, and basked in the warmth of that surprising serenity.

By the time tea was over, I was ready to face once again the uncertainty—and the inevitability—of the surgeon's knife. But to this day, I don't think Salvatore realizes the peace he brought that morning—the peace that forever destroyed my terror of coma and separation from God. Where there was despair, he brought hope—for a lifetime. For eternity.

Survival Rule #26:

No one—not one person—is meant to go through a cancer experience alone. Seek wisdom. Seek comfort. Seek peace. As a child of the Universe you have not only the right, but the responsibility to search for nurturing. Truly seek answers and truly listen when they come, whether from the clergy, loved ones, counselors or even chance remarks from strangers. You will know when words are meant for you and your healing.

XXVII

MOUNTAIN

*"Never measure the height of a mountain until you
have reached the top. Then you will see how low it
really was."*

Markings

Dag Hammersjkold

The Desert Clan arrived—my father from Tucson and my
brother Patrick from Phoenix. The week of Thanksgiving they
came to be with me before and during the surgery. Our Irish-
Scottish-Welsh clan has always been strongly supportive during storms, as my dad calls any tough ongoing challenge. We
may completely ignore each other during sunshine times, but
in any rough weather, we count on one another.

Morris and I showed them some of the sights of Houston—
the city's incomparable architectural skyline, the Galleria, Rice
University, the Astrodome and the Summit and St. Anne's mis-
sion-style Church among them. My brother Pat was most taken
with the deep fall colors of the trees, which were deeper and
richer than in years past—conditions had been just right the
previous year to create vivid burnished reds and golds. They
reminded Daddy of the autumns at Fort Apache, but this year
their beauty only reminded me of endings.

We did some early Christmas shopping and at all our

meals talked of family and old times and laughed as though there were no coming turmoil. We had only one tough moment.

When I wanted a beer "to calm down a little" before reporting to Houston Northwest Medical Center, both my dad and my brother "clouded up and rained all over me"—to use my dad's phrase—creating their own storm. For just a short time the ugly world of cancer was eclipsed by the world of evil spirits.

"Whatever you do, you remember this one thing—No matter what mountain you've got t' climb, what storm you've got t' face, a drink will only make it tougher. Not easier, not better, not ever. You remember what I tell you."

I listened. And I remember to this day, but at that precise moment, despite my father's admonitions and despite the peace I had encountered with the words of Salvatore and the young man at Corpus Christi, I still thought a beer or two—or more—would help me walk through the doors of that hospital yet one more time. Especially since all the tests and three doctors had diagnosed malignancy.

When I finally walked through those hospital doors stone-cold terrified, two days before Thanksgiving. I felt I was entering a deep ominous cave, a black hole opening in the side of an unscaleable mountain—a black hole from which I might never emerge. God only knows what "nightmare fighters'" I'd find within . . .

*   *   *

I awoke to my brother's loving face watching me. He held my hand and stroked my face and said the words I had not expected to hear—"It's okay, my sister."

I touched my chest, felt all the thick bandages.

"It's okay," he said. "It was benign. They gave you a new chest."

He smiled, waiting for me to grasp the meaning, the unexpected reality of this words. "Benign" this time meant a subcutaneous mastectomy on my right side and reconstruction on both sides of my chest.

I just closed my eyes and wept and whispered, "Thank You, God" over and over. When I opened my eyes my brother was weeping, as was my son and my friend Kathleen.

My dad came to the other side of the bed, grasped my other hand and said, "Well, I tried to tell you, you silly goose." But his mouth trembled in spite of his smile and his eyes, red-rimmed and tearful, looked at me with great love and concern and relief. "Well, by God, maybe *now* I can enjoy Thanksgiving dinner!"

Later that night, in the earliest hours of Thanksgiving, I awakened with words spilling over from thoughts. I reached for the rolling hospital bedside table, a pen and paper and just as though someone were dictating to me I wrote down these words:

> *My Dear Lord God,*
> *How difficult the path that leads to you.*
> *How steep, how hard, how painful the climb.*
> *You called to us saying,*
> *"All ye who labor and are heavy laden,"*
> *and I did not know the meaning of the words*
> *when first I heard them*
>
> *This soul-crushing fatigue*
> *cannot result from mere labor.*
> *This smothering, suffocating burden*
> *does not equate to heavy laden.*
> *You truly are the Master of All*
> *— including understatement.*
>
> *It's good to learn I am a goat*
> *— "Capricorn-rising"—*

the striving she-goat,
Climbing, scrambling, stumbling, falling,
Unsurefooted, but, Thanks Be to God,
Stubborn.
Sheer stubbornness enables this
stumbling, scrambling she-goat
to scale your slippery sheer cliffs
Of Overcoming and Love.

Now, in reality, I'm not "Capricorn-rising" at all. That label came from an amateurish and extremely inaccurate young astrologer in Tucson just before I came to Texas. He was as adept at astrology as I am with poetry, but the image seemed to work with the subject, so I just kept writing.

And yet, no sooner did I sense the awesome summit
than I slipped and fell again.
This time plunging headlong
to the base
to be broken
wholly
and ground into dust.
Until finally, even I
began to cry The Why? of it.

The Answer came—
Stubbornness and striving alone
cannot bring thee to Me.
Only tears from your Loved Ones
mixing with the faltering, faithless dust of you
can reform your clay.
Only their prayers to me
can lift you and show you
your New Way.
Reach out now! Can you?—

Say "Help me." Will you?
O stubborn, prideful one.
"Patrick, my Brother,
I am reaching.
How beautiful your outstretched arms."

"Salvatore, my Brother,
Please help me."
The difficulty in forming the words
dissolved in the selfless grace
of your Giving.

My dear Lord God,
Thank you for my brothers,
Patrick and Salvatore
and Daniel and for all my loved ones.

Thank you for my sisters, Kathleen,
Elaine and BeBe
and for all those who brought me
Your Hope and Your Care.

My painful desperate scramblings
Over the precipices
Have given way to peaceful pathways
and joyous acceptance
that you meant it when you said.

"Trust Me—
Trust Me—
for My Yoke is easy
and My Burden is Light . . .

"If you have Faith
and if you have Love."
My Dear Lord God,
I do trust You now—
in Life and in Death—
I Love You with my Whole heart,

> *Finally,*
> *Sharon*

Survival Rule #27:

Some mountains were never created to be scaled alone. When my brother and I were growing up our dad taught us many games which only ended when one of us yelled, "Calf rope!" meaning "I surrender."

As an adult fighting catastrophic disease, there comes a time when it is self-defeating to say in our childish manner, "I can do it all by myself." At these times the most healing words one can utter are "Calf rope!"

We know that Christ in his agony surrendered his will to God by saying, "Father, into your hands I commend my spirit." At some point in our lives we must be compelled to make the same life-changing decision—admit our absolute dependency on God and on our loved ones, father, mother, sister, brother or friend. Realize that it may be a gift to them to simply tell them, "I need you. Please help me."

Don't worry about repaying their kindness. The ultimate way to repay them is to help someone in need further on down the road.

XXVIII

SILENCE AND SOLITUDE

. . . I am going to lure her
and lead her out into the wilderness
and speak to her heart.

Hosea 2:14

The Jerusalem Bible

Sarita, Texas 1980—

A smiling, almost toothless Mexican viejito greeted me at the gatehouse. "Hola! Hola! Bienvenidos, welcome. Bienvenidos a La Parra."

He unlocked and swung open the white iron gate that led into La Parra Ranch, the second largest cattle ranch in Texas, adjacent to and over-shadowed only by the famous King Ranch. King and Kenedy were partners—the King Ranch was inland, while the land of the Kenedy Ranch ran along the south Texas coastline. Sarita Kenedy East, the sole heir of Miflin Kenedy, King's partner, had left her ranch mansion along with 1,000 of her several hundred thousand acres to the order of Oblates for a house of prayer.

First a private family ranch, La Parra later became St. Peter's Novitiate and still later a refuge for those, like me, burned out by too much life and death. Thank God, I was finally here. I was bone tired, soul weary.

I waved to the viejito and drove down La Parra road wishing I'd gone with friends to the Caribbean instead. I'd had my chance—Casa de Campo in the Dominican Republic and all the sunshine, hoop-la and gala nights of an international pro-am golf tournament. I had the desire, too. I just didn't have the strength. And I was sick of people and their endless prattle. I was almost sick of living. Depleted and depressed by chemicals and therapies and surgeries, exhausted mentally, physically, and most of all, spiritually, I needed a respite, a time a part, a healing time.

It was then Salvatore gave me his Christmas gift—an entire week at Lebh Shomea House of Prayer in Sarita. "Lebh Shomea" [pronounced *leb sho-may-ah*]—"Listening Heart" in Hebrew—seemed like a good name for a place that practiced silence and solitude.

The drive was exhausting and long—Huntsville to Houston, west to Victoria, south to Refugio to Kingsville and then here to La Parra, turning left at the single blinking yellow light in Sarita—about seven hours long. My little silver Grenada performed great. My father had given it to me two years earlier as an incentive to get well. As he handed me the keys he walked me around to the back of the car and pointed to the license plate—"TLW-099"

"That stands for 'The Long Way—99 Years.' Do you hear me?"

I heard. I just hadn't expected to do it all in one day. I slowly drove the last three or four miles to the main compound between strands of barbed wire that fenced in herds of cattle, mostly Hereford, and did not fence in wild turkeys or white-tailed deer that occasionally scurried and bounded in front of me, through, under and over the wires, disappearing into the surprising stands of grapevines amid the oaks and mesquites—surprising until I remembered that "La Parra" meant grapevine in Spanish. Just past a massive, rough-hewn wooden cross with a "crown" of barbed wire nailed to the top, I rattled across another cattle-guard and saw a huge white antebellum mansion surrounded by several white frame buildings and rough barns.

But that was all I saw. I saw no human. I parked my car and looked in all directions and saw no one. I walked all around and no matter where I searched I could find not a soul. It was eerie, spooky, not unlike Thomas Hardy's heath or even a Nancy Drew mystery from my youth. To augment the eeriness, the wind blew strongly, steadily, moaning around the eaves of the big, old house and surrounding bunkhouses and through the trees, nosily flapping the fronds of the numerous palm trees.

"Hello?" I called again and again. No one answered. Not a sound, just the wind and the palm fronds slapping each other. Finally, after knocking on a couple of doors in the bunkhouses and disgruntling two guests, I found someone in the basement of the big house, in an enormous kitchen filled with stainless steel.

She was a very tall, solemn someone and all her colors were strikingly mismatched. When she came closer to greet me, I was surprised to see she was only my height, around 5'8", but she seemed much taller for she was angularly thin. Dressed in no-nonsense polyester slacks, tailored shirt and sensible oxfords with soft silent soles, she had a narrow, delicate face, and her slenderness chiseled her features. She was pale to the point of whiteness. So this is what a "whiter shade of pale" looks like, I remember thinking. Her blonde hair, lightly laced with gray had been closely cropped in a style common to nuns and models and her eyes were of the palest ice-blue. One pupil seemed slightly larger than the other, like a minuscule ink-stain spreading around the iris, which only made the blue of her eyes icier. A visage severe, stern in anger, or even in response, I thought, but the minute she smiled hello, warmth melted her features into welcoming grace. She even laughed—chuckled—

Sharon Wanslee

heartily, although quietly, at my humor attempts as she guided me through the mansion, Roncalli library and the bunkhouse where I would stay, explaining the minimal rules. And when she laughed, her eyes sparkled electric blue and her cheeks were tinged with rose.

This was Sister Maria—director of Lebh Shomea—Sr. Maria Elizabeth Meister from Nebraska. I was to discover later that despite my immediate first impression, she had a most playful, happy spirit and loved to laugh, which usually prompted her to tip down her chin and cover her mouth with her hand so her chuckle wouldn't travel far in this silent realm, a gesture that made her look more like a mischievous school-girl than a directing nun.

As we walked through the mansion, the one-time splendor of its thirty rooms surprised me. The austerity of the dining room and kitchen on the basement level did not prepare me for the quiet opulence upstairs. Whispering, Sr. Maria pointed out rare books lining the custom-made glass—enclosed book-cases in the library on the second level, the lovely chapel at the north end of that floor, explaining that Sarita had her own chapel in the master bedroom suite on the third level, in addition to Sacred Heart Chapel, actually a small church, found at the east end of the driveway.

I kept whispering, "Oh, wow!"

I didn't see any of the third floor during that first visit. Sr. Maria admonished me not to enter there as all the bedrooms were occupied by visiting nuns.

What she didn't point out, but I couldn't help but stare at, were the custom-built breakfronts filled with exquisite antique china and silver services in the expansive formal dining room, the enormous crystal chandeliers and lamps, and the heavy antique furnishings, all accented by the obviously custom-made wall-to-wall powder blue Oriental carpet, the design of which outlined each piece of furniture. What astonished me most, however, was an enormous canvas n the formal living

186

room wall. Several other oil paintings that must have dated from the Renaissance were hung on that level, but this painting was the largest and the style seemed vaguely familiar. I peered at it more closely only to discover the name Velasquez. Another "Oh, wow!"—maybe I was looking at an original 17th century canvas of *the* great Spanish painter, Diego Velasquez in someone's extremely remove south Texas living room—out in the middle of somewhere between the Baffin Bay and the Mexican border. So impressed was I with the artist I have long since forgotten the subject matter of the painting itself. And it's not as though I could simply return and check.

It's all gone now. All that's left of the mansion's magnificence is the mansion itself. All that remains of its interior splendor are the vast expanses of highly-polished hardwood floors and the imported stained glass windows Sarita loved.

During one of my many return visits three years later, I was to discover her favorite window in the master bedroom's chapel. I stayed in the mansion that time, instead of a bunkhouse, in the bedroom called "Teresita," named after both saints—"Big Teresa" of Avila and "The Little Flower," Therese of Lisieux. This bedroom was really a screened-in sunporch opening off Sarita's bedroom. When I entered that room for the first time it seemed filled with Sarita's presence, but it definitely looked as though she'd finally decided to move out.

The enormous four-poster dark mahogany bed dominated the room. Immense it was and so massive as to be cumbrous, its bedposts were heavy and rotund enough to be mistaken for Doric columns. A three-rung matching mahogany sidestool stood handily by just to enter its domain. Just once I wanted to know what a bed like that must have felt like. I put one foot on the steps and looked down at the bare mattress, then back up at the Doric columns and couldn't do it. It not only felt too much mike trespassing, it looked too much like climbing into a tomb. I looked over against the facing wall and saw all the paintings—all those magnificent paintings, including the

Velasquez (not *the* Velasquez, it turned out)—wrapped, prepared for auction as though they were mummified.

I stepped down, took a couple of deep breaths to assure myself I could, and turned to look behind me. At that very moment, I understood more about Sarita. I saw what must have greeted her every morning of her life while living here at La Parra—a radiant masterpiece of stained glass, vermilion and cobalt blue, depicting Jesus kneeling in Gethsemane, above her own personal and private chapel. It gave a whole new meaning to Christ's admonition to go into your closet alone to pray. What a sight upon arising—and keening. So this is how the rich, religious people live, I thought. And die, I added, as I looked at all the stripped and packed belongings and mummified paintings once again.

I wondered if Sarita knew about the continued controversy following her death—the struggle over her land and its holdings, particularly its holdings *under* the land, a vast sea of oil.

I read later there was an intrigue involving New York factions, Texas factions and even a Vatican connection, all embroiled in a twenty-year-to-the-last-man struggle of greed and power.

One thing I felt certain of, however, if I were the one to die in this room, I wouldn't be concerned with it. None of it would matter to me. But that window would. I'd switch my pillows to the foot of the bed as I lay dying so I could see Jesus praying before his own agony.

Jesus is there still—praying—to this day while all else has been stripped, carefully packed and auctioned off. It now looks like a simple house of prayer—a very large house of prayer—and antique, art and rare-book dealers somewhere are happy.

An Essene would have been happy staying in my austere room that first visit. Sr. Maria led me to the center room of the bunkhouse nearest the library, west of the mansion, and opened the door into a room that more nearly matched my expectations of a house of prayer. Plain, barren and beautiful in its poverty, my room's furnishings consisted of a carved wooden crucifix, large, about a foot-and-a-half high, dominating the wall above a narrow, lumpy-looking little bed covered with a patched and threadbare white chenille bedspread, a heavy, dark brown desk, the type schoolteachers sat behind when I was in grade school, a squeaky desk chair and an old fashioned frayed and ugly colorless, upholstered platform rocking chair where I would sit each morning and evening watching cardinals in the tree outside my window.

"In this notebook you'll find a short history of Lebh Shomea and a map of all the walking trails—and a list of all the rules," Sr. Maria had finished her tour and all her explanations to my questions. "There really aren't all that many rules. The most important one, of course, is to observe the silence. Disturbing another's silence may be disturbing their prayer time."

I felt obliged to confess," Actually, that's the one rule that worries me the most. My father says I talk more than a two-dollar radio with a broken 'off' knob." I said that last part deliberately to make her laugh. She didn't disappoint me. And I was relieved to hear her say, and later to read in the notebook, that one could talk if it were important enough and brief.

The bell rang promptly at six. Silently people appeared as it from nowhere from all directions—the bunkhouses, the library, past the barns where the walking trails lay—filing silently one by one down the steps, past a myriad of cats, to the mansion's basement dining room. Dinner was simple—salad and sticky white rice with some kind of stewed meat sauce over it, all served buffet style along with tamales. I couldn't recognize the meat chunks. It might have been venison or even rabbit. It tasted terrible whatever it was. Maybe that explains why a large dish of salsa de chile verde was ever-present—a request of Fr. Kelly's, I learned—perhaps a constant assurance of flavor. Even smothered in salsa, however, my meal was left mostly untouched. Paper towels served as napkins and lazy-susan trays in the center of each round table silently served condiments throughout the meal. I felt dreadfully self-conscious throughout that first dinner. I just was not accustomed to sitting down to dinner without saying a word to my dinner partners. Even an occasional "Please pass the pepper," would have relieved the tension. My discomfort was such, I could not imagine enduring it over and over, every meal, every day for a whole week. In that awkward silence, I noticed seemingly everything about the nuns and priests and lay persons in that Spartan room. It's funny now when I think about how I thought they were noticing everything about me.

Survival Rule #28:

There is no true healing of the body unless the mind and the soul also become whole. And it is exceedingly difficult to find peace, health and wholeness of the spirit amid the din of our daily existence.

Seek peace. Seek solitude in a quiet corner—an empty church is ideal—if only for a few moments each day. In the silence answers will come.

XXIX

THROUGH THE LOOKING GLASS DARKLY

"'Curioser and curioser,' said Alice."
Alice in Wonderland
Lewis Carroll

Immediately following dinner, I met with Father Kelly—
Fr. Francis Kelly Nemick, administrator of Lebh Shomea—to
determine who would be my spiritual director during my
retreat. Fr. Kelly didn't talk much. This seemed only natural for
a contemplative, but as we sat together in silence I became
increasingly aware of how much of my life I'd engaged in
meaningless friendly-type chatter to put someone at ease, usually myself. I had to stifle words time after time. They just
seemed superfluous in this stark setting. Whole phrases would
form in my mind, melt in my mouth and vanish. I swear I
thought they trickled down to my stomach where they turned
to acid and growled audibly. I waited and listened to my stomach and observed this quiet man in blue jeans and white T-
shirt that made his skin, scorched from his ranch work in the
South Texas sun and wind, resemble dark terra cotta. His light
brown hair had been severely cropped in an almost-burr cut.
His spare not-too-tall frame seemed that of an ascetic, which I
believed him to be until I watched him eat tacos the following
Saturday night. Tacos are the fare every Saturday night at Lebh

Shomea. Preparing three or four at a time on his plate at the buffet table seemed ordinary enough, but Fr. Kelly **kept** preparing three or four at a time for three, four and then five times. I hadn't seen anyone eat tacos like that since two high school girlfriends and I would cook and consume tacos for hours until we ran out of tortillas. It didn't surprise me later to learn that Fr. Kelly was from Arizona, too.

"Sister Marie will be your spiritual director."

"Uh, yes," I nodded, relieved to hear words. "I met her this afternoon. She showed me around when I first arrived."

He looked a little puzzled.

"Tall, thin blonde lady" I offered, "from Nebraska?"

"no." The good father smiled slightly I thought. I couldn't really see his eyes behind his black horn-rimmed glasses due to lamplight reflections, so I wasn't sure. "No, who you met was Sr. Maria. Sr. Marie is a hermit nun from Newfoundland."

"I see," was all I said. But what I *thought* was that this was getting confusing. Marie?—Maria?—*Hermit nun*?! I was beginning to feel a little like Alice in Wonderland. Would St. Marie look a little like the Red Queen? Worse yet if she's a hermit nun, she'll probably more closely resemble Jonathan Winters' "Maude Frickart": iron-gray hair pulled back into a bun, square spectacles perched on the end of a rather bulbous nose, round plump, doughy body . . .

"You'll meet with her after mass tomorrow morning in Roncalli Library."

"I see," I said again.

Silence. Should I thank him?

"Thank you?"

"Thank **you**." he answered.

Silence. Am I supposed to go now?

"Good night?"

"Good night."

The minute I stumbled into my bunkhouse and fell on the bed, I dropped fast asleep—the day's drive had been so wearying. I slept so soundly, so leadenly, I couldn't figure out where I was when matin bells began to ring through the darkness at 6:25. But it sounded soothing and somehow familiar to be awakened by the mellow, rhythmic clanging of that big bell.

Mass that morning was short, simple and moving. Much of what is spoken or sung at other Catholic masses is celebrated in silence at Lebh Shomea. Fr. Kelly even raised the polished wooden paten—the Body of Christ—and the smoothly carved wooden chalice—the Blood of Christ—in total silence. I couldn't help but think of Teilhard de Chardin and his "Mass of the World," and imagined him celebrating in this silent and holy way. Fr. Kelly's face mirrored reflections of deep inner peace, but to this day, I don't believe I've ever seen such beautiful spiritual hands as the ones that held aloft those sacred wooden vessels. Working hands they were, slender, muscular and strong, burned red-brown—Michelangelo himself could not have found a better model to embody all the sinews and grace of hands both earthly and divine.

A young beautiful nun read the Gospel. She strongly resembled Genevieve Bujold, the French actress, but with short, wavy, pewter-colored hair, dark eyes and a very direct gaze. When she gave the homily, her look was so straight-arrow looking at each one of us, it personalized and empowered her message.

I liked the directness of her words as well: "repent means not so much to turn away from sin, as it means to turn **toward** God—completely. This always involves choices, and the choice is not always between good and evil. Often the decision is between the good and the **greatest** good."

Afterwards as I sat in the small sacristy off the chapel waiting for Sr. Marie, "the hermit nun," to appear, I again conjured up an image of a short, squat nun on the order of "Maudie"— gray bun, stainless steel spectacles, clumsy orthopedic shoes clumping right along into the 18th century with the help of a bent wooden cane clutched in gnarled and stiffened fingers . . .

"Sharon?" A soft voice called my name. "I'm Sr. Marie."

Imagine my surprise when I looked up into the face that more closely resembled Mlle. Bujold than Mme. Frickart.

Survival Rule #29:

Whatever your religion or non-religion, when you take the time to get in touch with the spiritual side of your nature, with all that is most sacred in your life, the healing in your soul cannot help but be reflected in your physical health.

XXX

LISTENING HEART

Give therefore thy servant an understanding
heart to judge thy people . . .

The Bible, I Kings 3:9
King James Version

There are moments so ordinary, quiet, and yet so significant that even as we experience them, we know they are life-changing. As soon as I sat down in Sr. Marie's office, I knew this was one of those moments.

We at first talked of Salvatore.

"I am **his** spiritual director here at Lebh Shomea."

"I know. He says you are most effective."

She smiled.

"He says you don't let him get away with anything. In fact, he calls you "The Pink Velvet Sledgehammer.""

In her surprise, her eyes and mouth grew wide and round. Then she threw back her head and laughed aloud.

I took a deep breath and began to relax. Prompted by her questions I began to tell her my reasons for coming and what I hoped to gain during my sojourn, and as I talked, I watched her listen. I could almost **hear** her listening to me. I found it difficult to take my eyes from her face, from her unbelievably profound and serene gaze, her soft, joyful smile. One of my greatest annoyances is to encounter people who do not really listen or who will not look at you as they do. "I need eye contact!" I always tell them. Sr. Marie seemed to make up for all of them.

Despite her eremitic life, her manner was easy and gracious. She was, in short, a surprise. She wore blue—a plaid skirt of varying shades of blue and a touch of rust, a sky blue sweater. Her shoes were a dainty pair of rust suede loafers, hardly a hermit's pair.

Her physical appearance confounded me, it's true, but it was her spirituality that first just surprised me, then captivated me. I became so mesmerized by her radiance that I felt I was looking into the most beautiful soul I'd yet encountered. There seemed to be a light shining from within her. At moments I was almost certain I was regarding the face of one of God's own angels. It was a little unnerving. Thank God she had a barely discernible lisp. An angel would have wings and a halo, not earthy rust suede shoes and a slight hint of a charming lisp.

"Is there a particular book of the Bible you'd like to study while you are here?"

In her presence I couldn't think of any. "Not really . . . I hoped, I mean . . . could you give me a suggestion?"

She just looked into my face, my eyes, and waited. Then she asked, "Is there a Bible **verse** that means a great deal to you?"

"Matthew 7:7. I have very few things of my mother's," I explained, trying to blink back sudden tears, "but I have her Bible and Matthew 7:7 was the only verse marked: "Ask and ye shall receive, seek, and ye shall find . . ."

"Why don't you start with the study of Matthew then?—and is there a writer or subject you'd like to pursue aside from the Bible?"

"I like Thomas Merton—in fact, if it hadn't been for his *Seven Story Mountain, and New Seeds of Contemplation* and the poetry of St. John of the Cross I would never have taken the final step to become a Catholic."

She was silent a while longer. She seemed to search my face for ways to guide me, and then with that light of hers still shining she proceeded:

"While you are here don't do anything until you are rested. Sleep—all day if you have to. But come to meals. You need strength. After you are rested—truly rested—begin reading. Each morning and each evening, for a thirty-minute period slowly read the gospel of Matthew. Then do the same with the book of Hosea. Savor the words, ponder them, re-read them. Then **listen** to what God may be saying to you through these words.

"Do not listen **for** what God might be saying, but listen **to** what He says to you.

"Then since you like Merton, read and study his *Contemplative Prayer* or *The Climate of Monastic Prayer*. You'll find them both in the library.

"Afterwards take long walks. Or ride a bike down La Parra Road. It's necessary to find a balance. But the most important thing is to rest."

So I did. I slept, I ate and slept a deeper sleep—what an Irish monsignor friend of my father's calls "a resurrecting sleep."

Another dinner—more chagrin. Mine the only chair that scraped loudly. Mine the only nose that dripped while I tried to eat and to sniff so silently—and unsuccessfully. What a terrible "Catch 22"!—the only way the food is half-way palatable is to smother it in salsa, but the salsa attacks my sinuses like strong horseradish. Consequently, if I eat, my nose runs—streams might be more accurate. I'm certainly not any "Miss Manners," but I'm not comfortable blowing my nose at **any** table, much less at one amid so many silent strangers. I tiptoed into the hall and honked a time or two, tiptoed back and tried to position myself at the table with no clacking, clanking, scraping or irritating noise of any kind.

Once reensconced, mine the only salad dribbling down a chin, and always, of course, when someone was watching. Mine the only sneeze in the group—why did it have to be so loud? Unobtrusive I'm not. Naturally the harder I try to be silent and graceful, the more loudly and clumsily I galumph along. I'd never make it as a nun.

I couldn't help thinking of the nuns at the Abbey in "The Sound of Music" as they sang—"How do you solve a problem like Maria?" No doubt I make the forgetful, noncomforming, noisy Maria look like Santa Teresa of Avila at her most contemplative. However, I am getting better with "The Silence."

Matthew and Merton started taking up more and more of my day. And when I felt strong enough, I began taking long walks along the meditation trails laid out just south of the mansion, accompanied only by my camera. The first day I made it to the resting place named "Golgotha," a clearing with a bench created for the purpose of contemplation. The next I traveled further to "Gethsemane," steadily progressing backward along a wilderness trail graced with dried reeds and rushes and grasses that rustled and sighed in the strong winds. It was lovely—and lonely.

One's sensibilities seem much more finely tuned here. Awareness not only of the spirit, the intellect or God—but awareness of all cycles of life and death is greatly intensified here at Listening Heart. Returning on the trail from Gethsemane I espied the tiniest caterpillar I've ever seen. It was no more than a half-inch in length, all orange and yellow fuzz, struggling to stay on the windy path and then almost immediately a bright orange butterfly flitted around me.

Predictable reflections on the cycles of death through transformation and resurrection filled my mind, when suddenly before me appeared "Death"—a large, disgruntled javelina boar snorting between enormous—and deadly-looking—tusks. He seemed most irritated that I stood in his path and might possibly be a threat to his herd. I slowly backed up to the barbed wire fence, climbed it not so gingerly and perched atop a fence post, a very slender fence post, to be sure, but a most appreciated one. I turned my back in feigned nonchalance and true nonaggression. I fervently hoped he would get the message. Waiting for his herd of probably fifteen to twenty javelinas of all sizes to pass through and under that wire fence took seven of the longest minutes of my life. The fence post seemed to get longer and sharper. Another interminable three minutes ticked by on my slow-motion watch before the boar decided to follow them, warning me with a departing snort.

Once my thudding heart calmed and my wobbly knees regained enough strength to climb down from my painful refuge, I found the sight of so many white-tailed deer hiding in the trees, gazing my way helped soothe my frazzled nerves.

But it was the sight of Sister Irma emerging from the oak thicket that made me laugh. She **looked** like drawings of the "Red Queen" in Lewis Carroll's *Alice in Wonderland*, which in itself is remarkable and funny enough. But this time the Red Queen wore lipstick—very bright and **very red**—on her very large lips which made her look like the movie version of said Queen. How odd! Even I don't wear lipstick at a house of prayer and certainly none of the other nuns do. She probably indulged in it to keep her lips from chapping in this incessant South Texas wind. She scowled so convincingly, I kept expecting her to suddenly point at me and shout "Off with her head!" I was tempted to photograph her to prove how real she was, but thought better of it. And I was given grace enough to contain my smile until I was much further down the path.

Over the years I've come to believe that often these moments come as a gift to counteract sorrow or loneliness. But this time it didn't work for very long, because I wished I could have laughed with friends, loved ones, about the cranky boar and the equally cranky Red Queen. Loneliness suddenly moved in like the Blue Northern, the Arctic cold front, that I watched approach as I turned back to the mansion—a tidal wave of dark and turbulent blue-gray clouds and cold wind rolling together into a veritable wall of storminess. With it came the impact of just how alone I felt.

I missed my son, my family, my friends. I missed the creature comforts of familiar surroundings, my music, my books, hot jasmine tea and my devoted, lovable Sam. And I'd only been here a few days. While I struggled the rest of that day to keep warm and keep quiet, I wondered how these contemplatives could bear their isolation for weeks, months, sometimes years on end.

I wondered if the Listening Heart of God understood my unspoken, unbearable loneliness.

Survival Rule #30:

Seek until you find your own "Listening Heart."

XXXI

ALL GOD'S CRITTERS

"As a doe longs for running streams,
so longs my soul for you, O God."

Psalm 42:1

Aside from my hour each morning with Sr. Marie, I'm not sure what proved to be more healing for me—spiritual studies or nature studies. One night I sat on the porch of my bunkhouse and watched the sun set the clouds on fire with its own color, and at the peak of the flaming, seven or eight white-tailed deer leaped across the field that lay between the sun and me. Two of the deer stopped close by to watch me, backlighted by the fiery colors, standing motionless for long moments before springing off again across the road to graze with the others. I never tire of these moments. Looking into their eyes is like looking into Timeless Being.

The deer and I watched each other for a long while each time I rode a fairly rickety black three-speed bike down La Parra Road. I stopped, as motionless as they, talking softly to them, telling them how beautiful they were. I've a feeling, however, unlike humans, they don't need to be told. They're too busy living and being fully deer-like. They merely gazed for long minutes before flicking their tails and bounding away. Before coming to La Parra, I'd never been within a hundred yards of a wild deer and now I've been close enough to touch scores of them. I wished someday I could be close enough to nurture as friend one of these mystical, half-divine creatures.

Throughout the day, every day, down that same road, eight or nine rotund wild turkeys scrambled through the brush, so round and fat I wondered how they could scurry so fast, much less fit through the fence. And every morning deer roamed freely and a herd of javelina rooted and grunted their way through the compound. I didn't know if it was the same herd that ran me up a fence, but I gave them wide berth. Most every one did. Maybe the permanent expressions of grouchiness sported by these critters makes them appear meaner than they really are, but the crankiest of all seemed to be the sows, the mama javelinas. As they grazed, their twin babies would suddenly dive under and between their mama's hind legs in search of their morning meal. The startled sow would jerk up her head from rooting, turn to scow at her rude offspring, snort, seemingly in disgust, then trundle off. The babies, now firmly latched onto her teats, would run double-time right along with her, heads still tucked under her spraddle-legged haunches, still sucking mightily. It was a grand snorting, smacking sight.

Late one afternoon while biking, I thought I caught a glimpse of a big blue bull! Son-of-a-gun! I turned back to see if my eyes were playing tricks on me. No tricks. He really was there about forty yards away through a fence clearing. A whole herd of exotic animals grazed there—some tawny, some really *blue*—all enormous and sleek, like no animal I'd ever seen before. This really *is* Wonderland, I thought. The only one not grazing was the biggest one. His head was up. Strangely enough he seemed to be a cross between a bull and a deer as he was much bigger than the others and appeared to be their protector. He watched me.

I stared, fascinated. He watched. I stared more. He watched ever more warily. I tried my deer-talk on him, even though I assumed he couldn't hear me—"Hello, bay, pretty boy, you're sooo beautiful . . ."—and as I watched him watching me a cold chill began at my scalp and crept slowly down my backbone. The look in "Blue Boy's" eye revealed a definite hostility as he bristled a few steps in my direction.

I lost no time in turning my rickety black bike toward the mansion and pedalled without regard for aching thighs pushing up and down hills. I skittered my bike to a stop in front of Sr. Maria's office and bunkhouse. I always sought her throughout the day for questions and answers and friendship, and I always made it brief.

"You were right to move on," she told me after I explained my haste. "those are the nilgai—a breed of blue antelope that Sarita imported years ago from India."

"*Antelope!* That big one looked like he was ready to charge me . . ."

"They usually shy away from people, but they can be hostile when threatened. If you had continued watching him, he could have become very aggressive."

I sat down.

Hand over her mouth, she laughed to see me so dismayed, even more dumbfounded than when I barely missed stepping on a large, bright green snake on the lower step of the library the day, before causing me to drop all my books and fall *up* the steps for yet another time.

As I parked my now fleet and trusty bike in the garage, I muttered to myself: Make a mental note, Sharon, antelope are not cattle; stags are not bulls . . . and, I smiled, *bulls* are not *cows*.

Remembering, I couldn't help but grin all the way back to my bunkhouse for "bulls and cows" always reminded me of the time after a Tucson rodeo when, as a very little girl, I asked my father about the difference between them:

"What did you say?!" my father asked aghast, beginning to tinge a definite shade of pink in front of our dinner guests, ranchers from Mammoth and San Manuel, who were also rodeo contestants in team-tying, and their wives. They seemed to find the question amusing.

"What's the difference between a bull and a cow?" I repeated as our guests found it more and more difficult to restrain their laughter and my father's face turned deeper shades of crimson until even I thought he looked funny. He scraped back his chair.

"Come on out here for a minute, Sharon. Excuse us," he said to our guests as he firmly grabbed my wrist and rapidly marched me out the front door to the gravel driveway. Then still holding onto my wrist he asked in a very low and serious voice, "Now just what was it you wanted to know?"

Totally baffled as to why it should be so difficult to get a simple question answered, I repeated the question slowly and patiently in a sing-song voice.

"Daddy! How can you tell the difference between a bull and a cow?"

My till-then omniscient father stood speechless. His eyes squinted in concentration and he kept running his free hand through his hair. When he wasn't searching my face, he was looking at the ground where he was scuffling his boot in the gravel and he kept clearing his throat. A picture of total helplessness, he looked calf-roped even to a four-year-old.

"Daddy, I just want to know—is a cow a girl and a bull a boy?"

"Yes. Yes! Is that all you wanted to know?"

"Yes, Daddy, but why'd you come clear out here to tell me?"

Kneeling down, he tousled my hair and gave me a great bear hug. I could hear the deep chuckles in his chest, *and as he laughed he looked and sounded as relieved as a condemned man cut loose from the gallows—just before the noose was clinched. Only years later would I understand why.*

He was an original, my father. He learned all about the birds and the bees from the bulls and the cows, and the stallions and the mares, and even the mean old boar he called "The Worser Pig."

Never long-winded on any subject, when it came time to tell my brother the facts of life, Patrick confided to me years later, my father paced and stammered and blushed and scuffed his boot again. Finally, he stopped dead in his tracks, jutted out his jaw, looked my brother square in the eye and ordered, "By God, Pat, whatever you do, you keep your levis *zipped!*" He emphasized each syllable by pounding two fingers on Pat's sternum. Then he turned on his heel and strode from the room.

Just as he learned about life through nature itself, so he learned about God. He just couldn't figure how there could be so much beauty and complexity around him without a great Creator. And the most beautiful of all sights to him was a herd of horses running free and playing in the wind, heads tossing, manes and tails flying. He was moved to the point of boiling anger each time he saw or heard of people hurting the earth or any of the wild creatures in it.

"By God, the stupid sorry bastards are just ruinin' it, ruinin' it for *all* of us," he'd say, shaking his head in total amazement that thee stupid people couldn't understand how connected everything is. "They oughta be horsewhipped!"

My great-grandmother taught him from the Scriptures and made him read the New Testament when he was a little boy on the ranch, and although I never saw him read from the Bible as an adult, I saw him live as though he did. And one little truck his grandmother showed him, he shared with my brother and me: if either of us ever had nightmares, our father would place a New Testament under our pillows to naturally—and super-naturally—disperse them. Our trust in him was such, it always seemed to work.

During mass the next morning, my mind wandered back to those long-ago days of innocence once again, and I reminded myself to tell Sr. Marie.

Fr. Kelly's voice interrupted my reverie: "An infantile perception of God's love is to think 'if I'm a good enough little girl or boy, God will love me'. That's wrong! God loves you, not because you're lovable. He just loves you—period."

A half-hour later, Sr. Marie admonished me to stop relying so much upon feeling. "God is just as much here in seemingly dark, dry periods as He is during times of consolation and visible signs of confirmation," she emphasized again and again.

"In the terrible dark times, that's when you have to rely on faith and the love of God."

Just like in my poem, I thought.

"Rely on faith, that inner realm of the spirit, and outward consolation will come when you most need it."

Later that afternoon I read Thomas Merton quoting from Isaac of Ninevah in *Monastic Prayer*:

> In the beginning we have to force ourselves to be silent. But then there is born something that draws us to silence . . . if only you would practice this, untold Light will dawn on you in consequence . . . After a while a certain sweetness is born in the heart of this exercise and the body is drawn almost by force to remain in silence.

All these words—Fr. Kelly's, Sr. Marie's and Merton's—were in my thoughts as I pedalled the old black bicycle alone and in silence the next afternoon. And no matter how fast I peddalled, I felt slowed down inside, more centered, calmer, less frantic. It seems I had been running, distancing myself from the medical nightmare, but now some small, but certain, sweetness *is* being born in my soul, drawing me more and more into silence. I watched the long blue-stem grasses blowing, swaying in slow undulations in the ever-present wind. I stopped my bike and leaned on the handlebars.

For many long moments, I watched the dancing grasses and listened to their hushed rustling. How I wished they could be seen from my window in the city. But it occurred to me, when I'm in the city and can't see the trees and the grasses, these beautiful grasses, that doesn't mean they cease to exist, anymore than God ceases to be when I can't hear or see Him.

Dear Father God, how strange to glean hope from your grasses blowing in the wind.

Survival Rule #31:

Nature's beauty and rhythms can bring us back into harmony of soul, with each other and with all living things. Find a place apart where you can experience Nature, wildlife and that part of your own Life that is *not* tamed, civilized and packaged appropriately for polite society.

Break away. Travel to "see a different tree." What you will learn about your Oneness with the Universe will be vital to your healing.

Your place apart doesn't have to be "spiritual," but it is crucial for it to be a definite "retreat" from all that is usual, normal and routine. The spiritual aspect will follow.

XXXII

A New Leaf

Thou canst not move across the grass
But my quick eyes will see Thee pass,
Nor speak, however silently,
But my hushed voice will answer Thee.

"Renascence"

Edna St. Vincent Millay

Departure day came. For the last time, I looked around my bunkhouse bedroom—the carved wooden crucifix above my lumpy bed with its threadbare bedspread, the desk I never studied at because it offered no view and the shabby, friendly old rocker that not only offered comfort but a great vantage point to watch the cardinals outside my window and the deer across the fence. Before packing up the last of all my belongings, I sat in the rocker one more time to copy in my notebook a last quote from Merton's *The Climate of Monastic Prayer*—a quote that seemed to sum up my life before and my hopes for the future:

> *Prayer is laborious when a man's heart is far away from*
> *him and God is far from the heart. Man's heart is far from*
> *him when it is occupied in superfluous cares or has grown*
> *cool in its religious fervor . . . God too is far from the heart*

*when he withdraws grace, withholds his presence and tries
the patience of the suppliant.*

*Prayer is devout (contemplative) when grace comes
quickly, when it fills the whole mind, when it is there before
it is called for, when it gives us more than we can ask or
understand.*

I closed my notebook and watched the cardinals for one
last time. Then I closed my eyes and felt the peace that per-
meated "Listening Heart." Thankfully, I didn't yet know that
my most contemplative, grace-filled days were still a few years
down the road. Nor did I know that the in-filling of grace
would be matched only by the outpouring of my grief.

All my preparations for leaving were nearly finished. All
that remained were mass at seven, then breakfast in the basement of the mansion, returning books to Roncalli and sheets
and towels to the laundry.

As I walked up the steps after breakfast, I intended to
return to my bunkhouse to put my suitcase and books in my
car before one last visit to Sacred Heart Chapel. And as I
glanced at my watch, I realized I'd have to hurry if I were to
beat rush hour traffic driving through Houston.

La Parra mansion's white gravel driveway diverged from
this back entryway, and my bunkhouse was down the path to
the right. Yet no sooner did I turn in that direction than I
stopped abruptly. I somehow felt compelled to turn to the left.

How odd, I thought. Puzzled, I turned back toward my
bunkhouse. Once again I felt compelled to stop. Once again I
felt turned toward the left. By this time I was totally disoriented, not to mention embarrassed. I glanced around to see if
anyone were watching this dismal state of indecision.

When my third attempt to travel down the path to the
right felt blocked and I felt not only turned but somehow
drawn down the path the left, I gave up. Maybe there was
some strange reason for all of this that I didn't yet understand.

And after taking only a few steps, I saw it—yet another exam-ple of Carl Jung's synchronicity—a big, shiny dark green leaf in the middle of my path. When I stooped down to pick it up, I saw that it was a most unusual leaf—one that had begun growing, had been eaten away by pestilence or disease, and had still kept growing from the same stem to form a whole, new and perfect leaf.

I cannot explain how such things happen. John Powell, the Jesuit priest and writer from Loyola University, says God speaks to us through our imagination. As I held that leaf in the palm of my hand, from somewhere deep within me, I heard, or more accurately, I felt, a voice that said, "Behold, I make *all* things new."

Trembling, I carried my new leaf back to my bunkhouse, to my room, now reached easily, unimpeded, by the path to the right. After searching for several minutes for the right pas-sage, I carefully placed the leaf between the pages of my Bible at Revelations 21:5 where "Behold, I make all things new," is written. Didn't Sr. Marie tell me that outward consolation would come when most needed?

Driving down La Parra Road in the little silver Grenada that my father had given me—with its special Arizona license "TLW-099" and its special message of "The Long Way—99 Years," I felt so grateful to God to have come such a long way. It's funny, I thought, here at Lebh Shomea, the more time I spent with wildlife, the more I felt I understood the scriptures. And the more I studied Merton and Matthew, the more I felt at one with nature and all living things. And it was from nature herself that I gleaned this gift of hope here in the Bible beside me—my New Leaf.

As the same Mexican viejito unlocked the gate, I looked down at this beautiful brand new gift and felt its message anew—All things can be made new again, right, God?— even me.

"Cuando regresa, hermana?" When will you return, sister?

"Muy pronto, señor, and muchas veces, si Dios me permite." Oh, yes, God, please permit me to return soon and often.

"Adios, hermana, que Dios te bendiga." Good-bye, sister. God bless you.

"Adios, señor, gracias, gracias. Hasta la proxima vez . . ."

As I drove through the gate, tears filled my eyes, not in sadness of farewell, but in gratitude for what I'd just heard myself say:

"Hasta la proxima vez"—until the next time. How many years ago had I replaced that beautiful phrase with my "Last-Time-Ever" mentality? Now suddenly here at the gate of Listening Heart, bidding farewell to this toothless viejito I realized "hasta" was back and with it my hope for the future.

Survival Rule #32:

Many years have passed since I found my "New Leaf." The more I have shared this story with others, the more I am convinced that this leaf is not really mine. Its message is for all of us—for you, in particular, who are reading these words at this very moment—"Behold, I make *all* things new" is the enduring promise. Grasp it. Believe it. Live it.

XXXIII

ANGELS OF MERCY AND THE COWBOY

*"I had fainted lest I had believed to see the goodness
of the Lord in the land of the living."*
Psalms 27:13
Holy Bible, King James Version

One thing my father told me wasn't true. Whenever he
spoke of loners—he was one at heart despite all his friends—
he'd always say, "You're born alone and you die alone."

A baby is not born alone, but into loving, waiting arms;
and no one has to die alone anymore. What he didn't know
was that we have angels of mercy now. A lot of people don't
know about them; I didn't until my father lay dying.

I call them angels of mercy, but they're really known as
hospice nurses. Hospice was first recommended for my father
by hospital nurses after a two-month debilitating illness, a loss
of forty pounds and exploratory surgery that revealed his "hep-
atitis" was, in fact, cancer of the pancreas. Unfortunately,
despite all the great strides taken in the treatment of cancer in
recent years, there was still not much the medical community
could do for this form of the disease.

Prognosis is bad—and swift. The surgery with its bypasses
would relieve my father's suffering for a while, his doctors and
nurses told me, but within a few months only the daily care

and supervision of a hospice nurse and team could help him.

So now Life had reversed our roles. It was now the daughter who knew the father was going to die. I could handle the old role better.

I dreaded the thought of calling the hospice. In order to relieve my father's suffering, I felt I would have to destroy any vestiges of his determined hope that he was "goin' to beat this thing." You only call hospice if the patient has a life-threatening illness with a prognosis of six months or less.

But his pain grew worse. Nothing alleviated his misery. Even the few pounds he'd regained after surgery were lost—he couldn't eat—and he was down almost 50 pounds from his once robust 190. It was like watching John Wayne waste away, only worse, because I knew and loved this cowboy.

And there was yet another problem. My cowboy father, who was known far and wide for being an all-around fair and honest man, was lying to his doctor. It just wasn't macho to admit to so much pain. So he suffered more and more in silence, hoping, praying it would get better.

It didn't. It was Time.

I drove directly to the hospice center without stopping to call, and it was the single most difficult drive I've ever taken by myself. I don't know when I've felt emptier, lonelier or more lost—arriving at the Tucson airport without my father's beaming grin to greet me or driving to St. Mary's Hospital to talk of his coming death.

So many times in the past I've gathered solace from St. Mary's garden. I even take comfort from a woven necklace made for me when a setting of five white stones, each one taken from this garden where my brother and I were born and where my mother died.

But that spring day I didn't take time to visit the garden and the white marble St. Mary. I just set my jaw and kept putting one foot down in front of the other along the path to the hospice, grateful for the Mexican bird of paradise in bloom and the yellow buds of the palo verde trees. Their familiar beauty seemed to make the path more approachable.

Once I walked through the hospice door, each staff member I met gave me comfort and new hope, not that my father could get well, but that his final days would be comfortable, filled with quality, meaning and dignity. And he would be able to remain at home. He hated the hospital—any hospital.

Joan Stemple, who would be my father's principal nurse, was working in the field that afternoon. I met her the following day—for lunch, I told her; for testing, I told myself—to see if she was right for taking care of my father.

While I waited for her in the restaurant, I thought about Daddy's last telephone call to me before I flew home to Tucson:

"By God, Sharon, I don't think I'm gonna be able to get it back."

These were his first words on the phone that day. He never did say hello; he'd just pick up our last conversation or his latest funny story. And he never said good-bye—he'd simply hang up.

"What makes you say that, Daddy?"

"Well, I went out to Oro Valley this mornin' and tried to hit just a few golf balls, and by God, I just *couldn't do it!* I just got no strength."

"Maybe you just need some new clubs," I offered, trying to keep it light and encouraging, all the while knowing it wasn't going to get any better. It rarely gets better when cancer of the pancreas is involved.

There was a long, long pause. Neither one of us could speak. I knew he was trying to get a hold on his emotions, and I was mentally packing and preparing to return to the desert, to his side, for the worst part was about to begin.

"Remember, Daddy, you've lost quite a bit of weight, so

lighter weight clubs might help. You're technically playing with an all new body."

He cleared his throat a few times, and then he laughed, "Ha! New body! Did I ever tell you that story about that ol' boy in the nursin' home?"

"I don't think so . . ." Whether I had or not, my answer was always the same, so much did I enjoy *his* enjoyment of the stories.

> *'Well, this ol' boy turns to this scrawny ol' heifer and says, "how 'bout me 'n' you takin' all our clothes off and streakin' across the front porch?"*
>
> *"'Hot damn!" she says. So they get after it, take all their clothes off and streak across the front porch and off int' the woods.*
>
> *'Now there were two real, real ol' timers sittin' and swingin' on the front porch, and after a while, one of 'em turns t' the other and says, "Did'ja see thet?"*
>
> *"'Yup."*
>
> *'Then they both swung back 'n' forth a time or two, and finally, the first one stops the swing and says, "Well, what was they awearing'?"*
>
> *'The other oldtimer shook his head real slow an' said, "I dunno, but it shure did need ironin'."'*

"That's my new body!" Daddy said.

I laughed through my tears and I know he did, too. When he hung up, I called the airlines . . .

The irony of his prolonged and painful illness developing, after his four bypasses in open heart surgery two years earlier, seemed particularly bitter to me . . . Why couldn't he have just clutched his chest one day on the golf course, playing in the sunshine with "ol' Doc Baldwin," his best friend and confidante? Dying with his boots on . . .

"Sharon?" Joan interrupted my reverie and held out her hand. I liked her immediately. Tall, nearly six feet, and trim, with light brown hair and enormous blue eyes, Joan's steady, direct gaze and soft-spoken manner, unflinching in the face of all my difficult, probing questions, won my trust.

My father liked and trusted her from the minute she took his hand and smiled hello. Our whole family learned to like her, trust her, love her. Her daily visits, and those of the hospice team—other registered nurses, a social worker and a young aide named Rick—became not only the highlights, but the guideposts, of our daily suffering existence. Joan was quick to understand that it just wouldn't be macho for an old cowboy to e tended by a female aide of any age, so it was Rick who lifted and bathed and shaved my father with as much gentleness and dignity as though he were tending his own father.

Each member of this team brought their own brand of comfort to my father's house, but it was Joan who always imparted a sense of quiet joy to our hearts. Often she met our needs—especially my father's—before they were voiced, and sometimes before we were aware of them.

But if I live to be one hundred and one, I will never be able to forget the Judas-traitor look my father shot to me when he first realized who Joan was and what her first visit meant. That moment will be forever freeze-framed in my memory by heartbreak.

Survival Rule #33:

Everything you have learned as the patient of a catastrophic illness can be utilized as a caregiver.

No one ever faces the death of a loved one without also confronting feelings about their own mortality. Accept this. Consult Chapter 19 of *Getting Well Again,* "The Family Support System," and work with patience and love in your nurturing of others.

XXXIV

THE SHEEPHERDER

"Where there is doubt, let me sow faith . . ."
St. Francis of Assisi

"Y'know, I probably haven't led a very good life . . . I mean by church standards . . ."

"What do you mean, Daddy?" We were sitting on the back porch, looking out over the Tucson valley, feeling the soft, desert breezes and listening to the gentle, sonorous tolling of the big windchimes.

He cleared his throat and looked somewhere off in the distance, his eyes squinting against the steadily increasing glare of the desert sun.

"Well . . . y'know, I never was much for goin' t' church or sittin' around listenin' to some o' them Bible-totin', psalm-singin' sonuvaguns."

I looked down and couldn't help but smile. True to form right to the end, aren't you, Daddy? And funny how at least three monsignors who could qualify as Bible-toters and psalm-singers consider you their greatest friend because of your refreshing honesty and earthiness.

"I'm sure your life reflects more caring for other people than a lot of Bible-toters who go to church every day, Daddy. And besides, one of the most important lessons Christ ever taught us was, 'Feed my sheep.'"

"I don't know what you mean . . ."

"He told Simon Peter—the one he was passing the reins of the church to—three times he told him to 'Feed my sheep.' And you've been doing that every day of your life."

"Slowly he shook his head. "Naw . . . naw I haven't," he said as though to himself. Then he looked a little puzzled. "What d' you mean?"

"Now I'm not calling you a sheepherder, Daddy, but literally and figuratively, you've been caring for the flock all your adult life—though it's difficult, I'm sure, for a cowman to think in terms of flocks and sheep. You always feed those who are down and out, who are hungry for food. And you always take care of those who are downhearted—by helping them with money or a verbal pat on the back, with words only you know how to say. When other people would wring their hands and worry about what they could do, you always acted."

he still looked perplexed.

"Do you remember all those little children who were abandoned in that garage apartment near our old house?"

He shook his head, totally blank.

"This was when I was a very little girl. I remember when the children were found, you were at work and everyone in the neighborhood it seems was wringing their hands and pacing and worrying about who to call, what to do, what state or county agency should be notified. Someone had the good sense to call you at work. I heard several people say, 'Mr. Wanslee will know what to do' . . . 'Clyde will take care of this . . . ' and all the while, Daddy, I *knew* you'd know what to do. I *knew* you'd take care of those little children and after you talked to them and hugged them they would feel safe."

He remembered. Tears filled his eyes and the inside corners of his dark, bushy eyebrows lifted as he furrowed his brow in that peculiar way of his that always gave away his tender feelings.

"Do you remember how you came home and mixed

together all those different kinds of Campbell's soups and took that big kettle to all those abandoned, hungry children, along with lots of bread and butter and cold milk—how you even spoon-fed the tiniest children, hugging them, holding them and wiping their tear-stained faces with your big grizzly-paw hands?

"Daddy, I think that's what Jesus meant when he said, 'Feed my sheep,' and it's most decidedly what he meant when he said, 'As you've done it to the least of these my children you've done it to me.'

"I watched you then and I've watched you all my life. You have been and always will be a model of caring for me. Each time I learned a scripture lesson, I always thought how you were *doing* what Christ said, and not just *saying* what he said."

Whether he was most moved by what Christ said or by what I said about him being my example, I couldn't tell, but he was quiet for quite a while with a look of pensive sweetness on his face.

He cleared his throat a couple of times to remove some of the emotion. "Y'know, one of the biggest problems I ever had with some of those church people was when they tried to tell me that there wouldn't be any horses in heaven." He looked as incensed as he did scared that this might be true.

"By God, I've known a lot o'horses that I'd a damned sight rather meet on that other side than some *people!*—sorry bastards that they are."

I couldn't help but grin. He always tickled me when he talked like that, especially because I knew he meant what he said. "But, Daddy, they really don't know what they're talking about! It says right in the Bible that when Christ returns, He'll be riding on a white horse."

"No kiddin'?"

"No kidding! Absolutely! It's written in Revelations. Now how can He ride in on a horse if they're aren't any where He's been?"

"No kiddin'? Can you find that part in the Bible?"

"You bet I can. You wait right here. I'll be right back."

I hesitated only an instant between the King James Version and my own Jerusalem Bible, thinking he'd get lost in all the "doths" and "rideths" of King James. When I returned and sat down with my Bible, his face had changed. He still watched quietly and sadly over the Tucson valley and the mountains beyond, the inner corners of his eyebrows lifted again in that unbelievably wondering, vulnerable expression of his, but his eyes for the first time reflected tentative hope.

"Daddy, let me read this to you:

> *And now I saw heaven open, and a white horse appear; its rider was called Faithful and True; he is a judge with integrity, a warrior for justice. His eyes were flames of fire, and his head was crowned with many coronets; the name written on him was known only to himself, his cloak was soaked in blood. He is known by the name, The Word of God. Behind him, dressed in linen of dazzling white, rode the armies of heaven on white horses. From his mouth came a sharp sword to strike the pagans with; he is the one who will rule them with an iron scepter, and tread out the wine of Almighty God's fierce anger. On his cloak and on his thigh there was a name written: The King of kings and the Lord of lords.*

As I read, his features crumbled. His chest heaved with silent laughter and sobs and his eyes and mouth laughed and cried at the same time. I held his still-strong, bear-like hands in mine and laughed and cried with him. We didn't speak. We were both lost in Daddy's vision of heaven—Daddy's *new* acceptable vision of heaven.

Survival Rule #34:

A patient needs to feel free to express any and all fears and emotions—both positive and negative—without fear of censure. Remember your own moments, days, of feeling alone and isolated, and do for the patient what you so desperately needed someone to do for you—listen quietly, understand and offer comfort and strength.

XXXV

RAINBOW

"Where there is darkness, let me sow light . . ."
St. Francis of Assisi

I wanted Time to rush on so Daddy wouldn't suffer any more. And how I wanted it to stand forever still so he would not leave us. He was sleeping off and on that morning. The only sounds were the distant, deep rumblings from the thunderclouds in the valley below us, and the wind creating original playful rhythms with the chimes right outside the open window.

I stepped outside to the porch to watch and feel and listen to the wind play.

"Sharon?"

I mentally kicked myself for not being right at his side when he awakened.

"Yes, Daddy—I'll be right there." I hurried in and sat beside him as he drank a few sips of Gatorade. As he lay back against the pillow, he grinned—"You know, Sharon, it's true— Old age is not for sissies."

How I loved my father's great humor, strongest when pressed down and out by sorrow or tragedy. I looked back out at the Tucson valley just in time to see an enormous, vivid rainbow arcing down from the clouds, seeming to touch down somewhere amid what passes for skyscrapers in the Old Pueblo.

"Daddy, look! A rainbow just for you. It's gotta be for you—it's framed perfectly in your big window. Wow, a rainbow!—symbol of God's promise to man. He keeps his promises with rainbows, Daddy."

There was that look again. Total vulnerability and hope all intermingled. We watched in total silence and awe—thankfulness—until that surprising rainbow melted into the rain.

Survival Rule #35:

As Kathleen taught me, the single most important thing you can do for a patient is the simple act of being there. Just *be there* in their hour of sorrow and greatest need.

XXXVI

THE YOUNG COWBOY & OLD BARNEY

*"Pity me that the heart is slow to learn
What the swift mind beholds at every turn."*

Edna St. Vincent Millay

"Would you like for me to read more about Merlin to you this morning, Daddy?"

I'd been reading—rereading—parts of Mary Stewart's *Merlin Trilogy* to him. Nothing relaxed him as well as reading about King Arthur and Prince Merlin of the line of Pendragon. He even shared something in common with Merlin—he was terrified of being buried alive. He seemed quieter than usual, more tense. The pain that Joan had been able to bring under control was coming on stronger, and the morphine sometimes gave him an expression I couldn't fathom.

"Not right yet. Run in there in my bedroom, in my third dresser drawer and bring me that story you wrote to me a while back."

It was a short, short story written for his birthday three years earlier, and I was very touched that he'd kept it so carefully. He told me he often read it, and I could tell this was so by the worn pages.

"Read it to me," he said.

"The Young Cowboy"
"Fill y'r hand, you sunuvabitch!"

A hundred times bigger than life—his repeatin' rifle in his right hand, his six-shooter in his left and his horse's reins in his teeth—John Wayne, fearless and magnificent, filled the screen. John Wayne at his best—playing Rooster Cogburn—confronting the nasty and nefarious Ned Pepper Gang in "True Grit."

God, how everyone cheered!—men, women and children of all ages. It seemed they'd never stop yelling, clapping and stomping their feet in sheer joy while watching the Good Guy get all of those dastardly Bad Guys, all by himself.

And I, a grown woman of twenty-six, sitting with my six-year-old son by my side, tried to cheer and clap my hands, too. But my cheers caught in my throat and my hands stopped in mid-air and fell to my lap. For during that famous slow-motion sequence as Wayne charged across that valley, and man and horse became one entity, one smooth flowing motion, I wasn't seeing John Wayne or Rooster Cogburn any longer. I was suddenly back in another valley, watching another cowboy and his horse— Captain Sixteen—become a symphony of speed and grace in sight and sound. I was back sixteen years [when I first saw the film] to that summer when I was only a gangly, snaggle-toothed ten-year-old fifth grader, sitting astride my Pinto pony, Sailor, out in the middle of the hot Tucson desert.

I was sitting and watching while big, powerful Captain Sixteen galloped furiously and fast right by me and Sailor again and again raising big swirls of dust. And as he galloped, the Cowboy jumped on and off him as easily as if the Captain had been a stationary fence post instead of a fury of motion.

At least two different times, the Cowboy ran up behind

the horse and at the exact instant he slapped him on the haunches with both hands, he vaulted into the saddle—so easily, so perfectly, the Captain never broke stride or even lifted an ear.

Man and beast moved together with one mind, one motion, one very special grace that day under the blazing Arizona sun. Aside from the movies and the rodeo arena, I had never seen anyone trick-ride, or just "plain ride," like that before. And even in the movies, I never saw anyone ride so smooth, so . . . so . . . natural-like, except maybe Ben Johnson or the Range Rider on TV. But this Cowboy was real life right in front of me and my pony.

I never said a word while that Cowboy rode. I just sat on my pony, wide-eyed, silent. I was afraid the private rodeo would stop—but more than that I was afraid of destroying the most magical moment of all my ten years— a time apart, a time transformed, a time when the Cowboy and the desert and the horse and the sky and the mountains and all of life moved to the same heartbeat. A time when I first understood the Cowboy's love of horses, of the land, of Life itself.

Years later, when I reminded him of that day and told him of my impressions, the Cowboy's response was typical: "Hell, daughter, did ya think I was born old?!!"

No, Daddy, I don't think you were born old. I think you were born very, very young—younger than all the pain and younger than all the fear and younger than all the hate this old world seems to inevitably dish out. You were born young and joyful and—despite all the bad guys and a dragon or two—you're still young and joyful and very loving and kind. I love you for teaching me to respond to Life in the same way.

"Fill y'r hand, you sonuvabitch!"—John Wayne fighting the Bad Guys in the Black Hats. My father, a hun-

*dred times bigger than Life, fighting the dragons, his own
and everybody else's, forever the Good Guy in the White
Hat—and always, always to me the Young Cowboy who
taught me to love Life.*
 HAPPY BIRTHDAY, 1981, DADDY—
 I LOVE YOU,
 Sharon

We were silent for the longest, dearest time, my cheek resting against the still powerful hand that grasped mine.

"God, I love horses," he said after a while. "Y'know, there are horses from the ranch I remember—*t' this day*—I can't think about 'em without tearin' up. In those days I think we all felt that way." He waited for another long while, as though the effort of memories was just too much for him.

He cleared his throat a couple of more times, and then he said, "Pecos Higgins worked on the ranch and he liked to write stuff. One night he sat down at the kitchen table real late one night and wrote about his favorite pony. Run get somethin' to write with—I bet I can remember most of it."

When I returned, his far away look made me think he was really seeing Higgins sitting at the ranch's kitchen table penciling his poem. I waited in silence until he was ready.

"Called him 'Old Barney' but it could be about any number of horses I've known. Write this down—"

"Old Barney"

*He was just a Spanish pony
That roamed the Rocky peaks.
He grazed upon the mesas
And he watered from the creeks.*

*He was known among the cowboys
As the kind they liked to ride,
'Cause he had Miss Wild Cow's number*

On any mountainside.
When the bushes went t' poppin'
And the dust began t' boil,
And the mallies went a-rollin',
Old Barney quit the soil . . .

"Then somethin', somethin, somethin . . . I can't remember a couple of verses here, but—"

Now when we wrangle horses
Out in this wild cow land
There's a little bay that's missin'
That wore a Spanish brand.
And when my time is over
And I cross the Great Divide,

His voice caught for just an instant, and I held my breath in sorrow—

I'll always call for Barney
When I want to take a ride.

"Y'know, Sharon, there's only one thing I ever thought was as beautiful as a herd o' horses, prancin' and tossin' their manes and tails in the wind—and that's a bunch of beautiful women twirlin' in pretty dresses, clickin' their high heels and tossin' their long hair. One always reminds me of th' other."

He closed his eyes for a while and just as I thought he'd dropped off to sleep he asked, "Does Morris have a gun?"

"No, Daddy, he's mostly into boats and skis."

Here it is, I thought. He's realizing how near the end he is and he's starting to give away all his prized possessions. Just the day before he'd given all but two of his golf clubs to his brother, my Uncle Bill. The other two he'd given to me.

"Go back in there in my bedroom and bring me my gun.

It's in the drawer of the headboard.

Countless times throughout the years I'd brought him a gun for cleaning, polishing, checking, so dutifully, sadly, unquestioningly I held out the weapon, a 38-revolver. I was surprised to find him seated, grasping the side of the bed.

He seized the weapon eagerly. I stood by and watched, trusting. At first I was sure he merely was emptying shells from the chamber, as he always did before examining or cleaning a gun. Slowly, too slowly it dawned on me that he was struggling for the safety catch—it took a long time for my mind to believe what my eyes were seeing. Stunned into a stupor, I managed to whisper, "Daddy . . . Daddy, I think you'd better give me the gun." I gently reached for it.

He pulled it sharply back to his chest, as if he were jealously guarding a once-in-a-lifetime poker hand. I tried to grasp it, more firmly this time.

Superhuman strength stopped me. This enfeebled man, who unaided could barely lift his head from the pillow or his arm from the quilt, suddenly catapulted from the bed, frantically fumbling with this malignant carrier of death. His hands shook fiercely from the adrenalin-charged effort and from the morphine.

Where was *my* strength and *where* did he get all this brute force? So strong, so strong—the strength of *ten* men!—my God, overpowering . . . this *can't* be happening!—My God, he's trying to kill himself and dear Christ, he's trying to shoot *me first!*

"Daddy! *Daddy, please!*", I looked into his eyes. Oh, God, his terrible eyes. I can still see there the depths of murderous hell.

"Jesus, help me . . ." I whimpered. "Help!" I managed to shout. "Someone, **anyone**, help me—Please help me!!!"

There's no one to help.

For several long moments we struggled as Time and my breathing stood still. Suddenly, with a new surge of ungodly strength, he jammed the searing coldness of the gun barrel against my cheek and held it.

I stopped moving. I became deathly still and distant as the gun burned like dry ice into the side of my face. Part of me seemed to observe from the corner of the room, somewhere near the ceiling, directing. All other parts seemed incapable of movement, except for the thudding heart that filled and shook my chest.

"Struggle. STRUGGLE!" a voice shouted at me.

"Fight! You must FIGHT!" the voice assured me or "you will surely die. You will both surely die!"

"Daddy! Daddy! I gasped. "What are you doing?!—for God's sakes, *Daddy!!!*"

Only silence and those murderous malignant eyes answered me as we continued to struggle.

"I . . . SAID . . . GIVE ME . . . THAT GUN!!!" The voice thundered and with the voice, *my* voice, my strength resurged. I wrenched the loathsome thing free from his living grip of death. Immediately he collapsed back upon the bed—beaten, broken and still silent.

As I staggered from the room, securely grasping the gun with both hands, chills shuddered through me, my teeth chattered, but I didn't cry.

Ah, God can You hear me? Can You see me? Did You see my beloved Daddy try to blow my brains out, for Christ's sake?! In leaden slow-motion, I emptied the shells from the chamber and bitterly contemplated how I had just saved my father for a slower, more excruciating suffering.

As I hid the gun, my knees buckled and my heart broke.

Survival Rule #36:

Understand that morphine and other pain-killing medications can alter a person's mind and emotions, their entire persona. And it is not at all unusual for men of great strength of mind and will to try to take their own life upon suffering their own terminal illness. Feeling totally out of control of their life, they "take control" of their own death.

XXXVII

PASSION PLAY

"When . . .
the great star early droop'd in the western sky in the night,
I mourn'd, and yet shall mourn with ever-returning spring."
"When Lilacs Last in the Dooryard Bloom'd"
Walt Whitman

His death bed emerged from a king-sized sofa. He liked it better in the living room surrounded by his favorite possessions—all his books of history, biography and the days of King Arthur and Prince Merlin in wall-to-wall shelves, my grandfather's spurs, all his summer and winter Stetsons and coiled ropes hanging from the expanse of elk horns his old friend, Carl martin, had given him, and of course, the view. By night he could absorb the multi-colored shimmer of Tucson lighted below him in the valley, and by day, he silently observed the unending parade of desert animals and birds that made their way to the perpetual watering hole he'd had built. Roadrunners, woodpeckers, mourning doves, cactus wrens and the pigeons from his garage, along with timid cottontails and big, bold jacks, lizards, snakes and any stray dog or cat, sooner or later found this tiny oasis. I once saw a coyote furtively approach and drink in the middle of the scorching summer's darkest hours.

But on this, my father's darkest night, he was unaware of the animals or the view. We all were. Our eyes were on him and his agony and he was looking at something we could not see.

It was the Saturday night before Holy Week. There must have been fifty to sixty people present, almost all family, many surrounding my father's death bed, many more spilling over into the desert.

Those my father loved most encircled his bed, three and four deep. I knelt at the foot of his bed, sometimes stroking his feet. My brother Patrick with tears streaming non-stop down his face, held our father, supported him as he struggled upright over and over—trying, trying to take in air with desperate, rasping breaths that were terrible to hear and crucifying to behold.

Father Tom sat among us, a tower of godly strength. He had driven across the city to give Daddy last rites—again. Maybe for some, last rites are not enough. Maybe some need them again and again as the panic rises. No one had ever before been able to impart any peace of God to my father, and I'm sure Fr. Tom succeeded because he embodied the power as well as the love of God. My father's peace had always been what Fr. Tom described in his Irish richness as "of the airth." Now his peace, both earthly and heavenly, was gone, and for this reason, I begged the good monsignor to stay with us.

Music helped. It had always relaxed my father—especially easy-listening music stations. But that night the music ran out and an incongruously dry and rambling talk show began. I think it was about school boards. My father became even more restless. He never did like school-board meetings.

I changed the FM tuner to what I thought was a light classical station. Beautiful, celestial music filled the room, ethereal enough, I thought, to help Daddy storm heaven's gates. No sooner was I seated again at the foot of his deathbed than it began—Christ's Passion Play on the radio. It was the day before Palm Sunday. Betrayal, suffering and excruciating death recounted as I watched the reenactment come to life—and death—before me.

My father lay with arms outstretched on either side, and as he agonized his way to a sitting position for more air with the help of my brother and step-brothers, his eyes sought mine. The more he struggled, the harder he warred against the treacherous body betraying him, depriving him of air, the more frantically he battled to breathe, the more fully I knew the slow and terrible agonizing asphyxiation of Jesus.

Suddenly, explosively, the grief of it all shattered my heart, and with the breaking, a blood-curdling keening arose. It filled to overflowing all the silent, waiting spaces of the room, and I later learned, terrified all the silent waiting souls within the hearing.

Fr. Tom gathered me into his massive embrace and held me close until my wails died, dissolving into silent, streaming tears. A long, long while passed before my brother pulled me from Fr. Tom's strength into his own. When he did, my face was smeared with red and Fr. Tom's black clerical shirt was drenched in blood. My sorrow once again spilled over into bleeding— another hemorrhaging nosebleed—the third one this week.

Hours passed, moment by undurable moment.

Through my numbness, there came a knowing—a still, small voice that told me the Time was rapidly approaching. As if lifted by the Dark Angel's unseen wings, I rose from the floor and marched determinedly into the front bedroom. I carefully shut the door and just for a moment allowed myself to lean back against it. I closed my eyes remembering how Fr. Bob Costello, the visiting Jesuit in our parish had taught us that sometimes we have to stand in the breach between God and man. Just at that instant, I was given words for the most powerful prayer of my life.

I planted my feet firmly apart, clenched my fists and looked heavenward as from the depths of my being came:

Do You call **this** merciful?!!

Please *take* him for Christ's sakes—

Take him in the name of Christ—

Amen. Amen. And ***AMEN***.

After only a moment's knowing stillness, a single strong heartbeat, my brother and step-brothers and aunts called out to me—"Sherrie, he's gone." "It's all over, Sharon . . ."

I already knew. I opened the bedroom door and walked out into a world no longer graced by my bigger-than-life father. I waited until everyone left the room. Some wept. Some merely looked sad. All of them looked lost as they kept saying, "Well, at least now he's peaceful." "How peaceful he looks."

I didn't think he looked peaceful. I thought he looked gone. Through my numbness, I felt relief. For several long moments I contemplated the empty form that had once been animated by my father's glorious, one-of-a-kind cowboy spirit.

Well, one thing's for sure, Daddy, I thought, you didn't get outta this one alive, but you sure got outta this loved! And one more thing. You were wrong! You sure as hell didn't die alone—there were at least fifty people with you when you died. And a big part of me died right along with you.

"I love you, Daddy," I said as I closed his eyes—for the last time ever. Then I slowly walked out alone into the desert under the cruel April sky.

The next morning, Palm Sunday, at the Desert House of Prayer in the Tucson Mountains where I was staying a monk wrote in silence on the blackboard of the retreat dining room:

Desert flowers struggle forth
once again to say
Tombs cannot end
Life.

Survival Rule #37:

Tombs *cannot* end Life or Love.

XXXVIII

ALICE, IN TRUTH

*I merely took the energy it takes to pout
and wrote some blues.*

Duke Ellington

Years passed. Throughout all that time of teaching CMT to cancer patients, I thought Anna would prove to be my most difficult student. But then there was Alice. Her life story portrayed more melodrama, more twists and turns and convolutions than most soap operas. In fact, she always claimed she'd never watched more than a few minutes of a soap. "Too tame," she'd say. Even "Mary Hartman, Mary Hartman," the '60's spoof of TV soaps, held no interest for Alice, who felt, in her own words, "totally bamboozled by life," especially by deliberate unkindness.

With here permission, I have read and quoted from her journal to piece together the memories of her life and their healing. She warned that:

> . . . in an era that exposes the atrocities of ongoing racial hatred . . . and that reveals practices of women in India burned for their dowries, and of African girls mutilated to "welcome" them into puberty and with sexual abuse and rape rampant in so-called 'civilized' countries in war and

in peace, the battering of one single soul may sound as a self-pitying whine. Yet because my experience was solitary, it was no less pernicious and insidious.

She stopped reading and grinned. "I just don't want this to sound as pitiful as Dolly Parton's "Coat of Many Colors." Alice always used humor to soften the harsh edges of reality.

Our class sessions were the ones I most dreaded. I thought she'd never have a most-needed breakthrough, and once she did, she'd need another and another. She was in her mid-thirties when she first entered the CMT program, and her repressors worked longer and harder than those of anyone I worked with—before or since.

She'd been a cancer patient—breast cancer, as so many of my patients—and she did everything she possibly could to be positive, active, forward thinking. But she made me start believing in the possibility that one *could* be born under an unlucky star. Her paintings revealed such anguished strokes, such mournful, angry colors for hundreds of paintings, I found it my biggest challenge to elicit more openness, more freedom of emotion to pull the pain from her soul. I continued to work with her with great patience long after the eight weeks were up. I wanted her to survive, and I was afraid her pain, her deep inner sorrow would kill her.

Over 1500 paintings splashed from her brushes before she uncovered the rage she felt toward her father. He'd taken Alice and her brother from their mother when Alice was but a few months old and her brother was five. Before Alice was three he remarried. And all the nurturing love and tenderness Alice had known from her mother suddenly was exchanged for the brutality, hostility and ridicule from the stepmother, a cruel parody of all the evil caricatures found in fairy tales.

This Ms. Hyde, who locked Alice in closets, slapped her when she was most off-guard with such force it send her senses reeling and her heart cowering, would suddenly metamorphose into a charming and chilling Mrs. Jekyll when anyone else appeared. Then when Alice grew too big to brutalize physically, the emotional battering began, so relentless *"it nearly crushed my soul,"* she said with such a haunting voice, I could feel her long-ago pain.

I simply could not understand how her father could take her from a loving mother and place her with such a harpy. That action, committed by the person she loved and trusted most in the world, stole her young life away. Not the worst paradox I'd ever heard, but a memorable one.

Alice grew up in terror. She never knew when the next battering—either physical or emotional or both—would begin. For example, one CMT painting session thrust her way back to another painting time. Playing with paints had been her favorite childhood pre-school pastime. Her journal notes read:

> *I became alive, absorbed, quietly joyful, each time I worked with the vivid, happy colors. Until that awful day my stepmother punished me for spilling a few—literally three or four—drops of paint on my child-size table. The punishment?—to gather all my beloved paints and brushes and small canvases and throw them into the trash.*
>
> *The only times I had felt more heartbroken in my life were the handful of times I had seen my mother every few years for just a few short hours and then had to leave her again.*
>
> *It felt like soul murder.*
>
> *How ironic I was given this gift of CMT, the healing instrument that requires one to stir up tempera paints and* make the biggest possible mess.
>
> *Unlike Perseus, my saving weapons against my own personal medusa became a paintbrush and a jar of paint. Instead of Hera's shield and Hermes' sword, these colorful*

instruments gave wings to my heart and mind.

The worst chapter in the saga of her young life was that each time she tried to tell her father what happened in his absence and what Ms. Hyde was really like, Mrs. Jekyll would follow with words that called the girl a troublemaker, a fabricator, an out-and-out liar. To her dismay, her father believed Mrs. Jekyll's twisted words. And that belief shattered all hope for the young girl. She learned that if she spoke out, complained of anything to here father or brother, Ms. Hyde would become even more vicious and vitriolic. Alice learned not to speak of what went on inside those walls ever again. She was five at the time.

I wanted to blame the stepmother, but upon hearing that unfortunate woman's story, I couldn't. She was after all only another victim—of abuse and abandonment. She vented the pain and rage of her life on the nearest subject at hand, which unfortunately, was her stepdaughter. Paradoxically, this same stepmother made sure she had dance lessons—ballet, toe and tap—and baton-twirling lessons, and insisted that the girl specialize in French and Spanish classes. Another paradox—she might be battered, devoid of any confidence or self-esteem whatsoever, but, by Jove, she would be cultured and graceful.

When almost all Alice felt at home during those formative years was fear and sorrow, the wonder was *not* that she shackled her emotions and lost the key; the wonder was that she ever found it again.

She rebelled once. It was in the fifth grade. She had accidentally dropped her hairbrush into the bathtub, creating a terrible clatter. The stepmother somehow took this as a personal affront, and flew into the girl with a terrible rage—hitting, slapping, beating, cursing, screaming obscenities—again. And Alice just couldn't take it anymore. She hit back. Just once. But once was all it took to unleash the years of anger pushed back and down. She hit back again and again and shouted, *I hate you - I hate you . . .*

She almost overpowered her, too, probably because the stepmother was so taken by surprise. Her attacker left for a moment. Alice caught her breath, hoping the worst was over. But, as she wrote in her journal:

> ". . . *the screaming Medusa was suddenly back, cursing, screaming, twice as strong and flailing a wire flyswatter with a ragged edge. Each time the cursed instrument slashed across me cutting into my flesh, I lost more strength and hope. She had won—this battle—but she never again tried to beat me physically."*

She lost herself in books—the very first full-length book she ever read was, appropriately enough, *Alice in Wonderland.* That convoluted, psychotic world of Carroll's seemed only too real to her—she felt she was already living with the Red Queen's evil twin. School was her salvation—she immersed herself in studies and excelled, and told herself it was okay that one part of her life was dreadful, because the other part, school, was such a joy. And through school and reading, Alice learned of others who had suffered much, much more—those who had suffered the atrocities of the Trail of Tears, of Black slavery, of the Holocaust; on the bottom shelf of the family bookcase was a pictorial essay book about World War II. She couldn't believe the suffering she saw depicted in those pages—the Holocaust and its victims—and no one came to help. It gave her a whole new perspective on suffering.

Her silence grew more profound.

Humor would be a saving grace for her. Alice constantly sought the droll, the humorous the outright outrageously slapstick, and the closest friends she maintained all throughout her life were natural-born clowns—kind and gentle—but clowns, nevertheless.

> *"My dad was redeemed," she wrote, "if someone or something made me laugh. And if I could laugh from my stomach, or better yet, from my toes, it was a great day—no matter what waited at home."*

Her own experience had taught her to be keenly in tune to the underdog. Alice found she absolutely could not tolerate the kids who beat up on the class hunchback or taunted the young Hispanics who had trouble with English. What seemed even more intolerable to her were the teachers who punished those same kids for speaking Spanish on the schoolground—or *anyone* with power abusing those without it. As silent as she remained at home, the more outspoken she became at school.

And day by day, the stepmother worsened. Abuse became more verbal, more hateful.

But the day of reckoning finally came. By some miracle, Alice's father walked in on the hatefulness. The stepmother, thinking he was at work, started yet another tirade against the girl, who had learned to just sit quietly and endure. Any word, any gesture, even any glance would only set off a more highly-pitched fury.

Her father stood there, one half of his face still covered with shaving lather, more lather dripping down his arm from the razor in his hand, his mouth agape, his incredulous expression mirrored the sickening realization that Alice had been telling the truth.

"Well, I'll be damned," was all he uttered.

But the pain and astonishment in his eyes said that in that single moment he understood everything she'd been trying to tell him all those long years. Finally. Alice was almost fifteen years old then.

The stepmother was sent away—for good—that very day.

The long years and the stepmother's efforts did not destroy the relationship between Alice and her father. If anything, from that day forward, a new bond formed between them—a

bond of friendship and renewed trust and humor—held firmly in place, no doubt, by remorse and forgiveness.

Alice learned to let it all go, to let it be, to forgive totally
and by so doing, to forgive herself—as she hoped to be par-
doned by others for her own errors, her own failings. She felt
strongly that all she had experienced had worked to deepen her
capacity to love and forgive and to nurture. As she wrote in her
journal:

> *I am convinced that everyone in that slow, sad
> drama—my father, my mother, my brother, my stepmoth-
> er—did the vest best they could with the insight they had at
> that given time.*

"I am grateful," Alice read aloud from her journal one
afternoon in class, "I recognized it all as a lie. There were people in my life all along the way—mostly, my wonderful, pro-
tective brother, teachers—one extraordinary high school counselor named Maria Urquides, in particular—one Sunday
school teacher, great friends, even great strangers, who were
kind to me—sometimes for long periods of time, other times
for just a single moment. Those people kept me going, kept
me believing in goodness and loving kindness."

After a long pause, she added, "I thank God for each of
them every day—and for puppies and big dogs and roses and
for anything that makes me laugh." And then she laughed
right out loud at the very thought of these things, possibly
from nervousness for revealing so much of her life, but mostly
from the sheer joy these things brought her.

She laughed again when she read from her journal about
how she grew up *never* wanting to marry. Later she decided *if*
she married, she never would divorce—she felt it led to too
much unhappiness, especially for children. But fate inter-
vened. She married—for ten years, had a son—and divorced.
She married again for six years and divorced. Five years passed.

The third time surely will be the charm, she told herself, as she married yet again—"For good," she told herself, the new husband and the old preacher. Yet ten years later, much to her surprise and devastation, she once again divorced. They wee each good men—the Schoolteacher, the Ad Man and Mr. Golf— three good men with flaws, of course; chief among them was the desire to make up for all the lost years of her painful, isolated childhood. They failed, not because they weren't good enough or strong enough, but simply because the only person capable of filling the voice in Alice's life was, of course, Alice.

Each time she found herself thinking her life just didn't seem to be going the way she'd planned, she thought of her son. She was fiercely proud of the child she bore in her first marriage, when she was 19. She raised him with great love and tenderness and Haim Ginott, the psychologist/author who wrote *Between Parent and Child.* Alice once heard him speak about chastising the action, not the child, and always treating a child with respect and dignity and it not only made more sense to her than other more complicated child psychology theories, it radiated with compassion. She bought his books and used his ideas and nurtured her son with all the tenderness she'd longed for as a child. As a result, he grew to be a well-adjusted, successful, happy young man, despite the upheaval in his mother's life. She and her son were not only parent and child, but good friends, which they are to this day.

Not only was Alice exceeding grateful that she did not perpetuate the abuse, she felt fierce pride and great accomplishment in the fact.

"I wanted to add a whole new meaning to that old saw— 'The buck stops here.' The buck—*and the pain and the lies*— stop here." She was never so sure of her success until the day her grown son said he had seen the film, "Mommie Dearest."

"What a crock, Mom!" he told her. "No one could treat anybody like that."

Alice just smiled. She waited for another day to tell him her own young life had been worse—much worse.

Alice worked through many damaging memories in her paintings and journal work, delved deeply into the healing of all her past, but she would always ruefully wish she had not perpetuated the pattern started by her father and brother of three marriages each. The only good she could glean from this situation was that of growth—"It forced me to grow—and adapt," she said. "If adaptability is the one of the hallmarks of intelligence, I must be nearly a bloomin' genius by now."

Then came the day when she couldn't bear to look back even one more time. She put away her paints and brushes for a while, remembering how her father replied to critics when he stopped attending AA meetings—"Well, I had the measles once, too, but by God, I got over 'em."

That's how Alice felt.

"It was time for moving on," she wrote. She'd gotten past all that pain. She'd gotten over it. *Thanks be to God.*

I know everything in her journal is true, for I am Alice. It's my middle name, borrowed from my Irish maternal grandmother. Alice means "Truth."

Survival Rule #38:

For the Abuser:
Get help. There are those who will understand your cry for help, who will accept you and set you free from the pain you carry that causes the pain you inflict.

For the Abused:
Find help for yourself. Find a method, some process or therapy that will lead you through understanding the pain of the abuser to ultimate forgiveness. Only then will you be healed.

And never, ever pass your pain on to others. The pain must stop with you. And you must grow through it.

XXXIX

THROUGH MY FATHER'S EYES

The former things have passed away . . .
Behold, I make all things new.
          The Oxford Annotated Bible
                    Revelations 21:4-5

For the first time ever I carefully unwrapped the 13" by 16" heavy wooden frame that held the best photograph of my father. I'd taken it three years before he died. In the photo he stands before a palo verde tree in the middle of his rock-lined circular drive in the foothills north of Tucson. He seems to emerge from the desert itself, and so he did.

As always he wears western cut clothes—with a fawn-colored corduroy jacket, the wide, soft leather belt with the sterling silver Zuni buckle, a pair of boots made from the hide of water buffalo. He'd had them for years and years, long before the phrase "endangered species" became a part of our lives. And despite the Stetson shading his eyes, I can still see the absolute steadiness of that brown-eyed gaze and the sweet half-smile that forever mirrors the tenderness of a father's love. Each time I look up at that photo on the mantle I swear I can hear him say, "Sure good t' see ya." It brings me much comfort now, a quiet sad joy and many memories, but before I could let it be part of my life again, ten long years had passed.

I can still see there the joyful tears shining in his eyes to learn that Campos had pronounced me "absolutely, positively cured"—fourteen years ago now, the same year I took the photograph. To commemorate this my father gave me a Zuni butterfly pendant. I wear it often, especially when it seems I've been existing for long periods in a cocoon, where nothing seems to be happening creatively or spiritually and it takes such courage just To Be—and suddenly once again I become aware I've been given wings.

This turquoise and silver butterfly—just as my butterfly painting—has become for me the symbol of a being who has discovered New Life despite the darkness and fears experienced in its enigmatic hibernation—or maybe because of them.

This photo also reflects the quiet amusement in my father's eyes when Father Tom and I reminded him of how we circled his wagon, disarmed him and drew him into the Catholic faith. Father Tom, Monsignor Tomas Cahalane of County Cork, Ireland, sent a message through me that he was coming after my dad.

"Tell him," this towering priest instructed me, "that the name Cahalane means *'ready for battle,'* and it wasn't long before my cowboy-father, desert son of a pioneering Mormon family, faced the battle and joined the good monsignor's army, thus saving our family the disgrace of having to line up and throw golf balls at his casket at St. Augustine's altar, as Fr. Tom originally prophesied.

Pleasure would have shown in my father's eyes to learn that I'd continued to devote time to cancer patient s— with my CMT course and with emotional and moral support. For years I wondered why I felt so driven to help them. There was, of course, the debt I owed because of my mother, and the gratitude for all that had been given me. What I could not realize at the time was that it had all been training, preparation, for during each of my father's stages of debilitation, it occurred to me I'd already been through the same process with George or Anna or Emma or Mr. Roberts—the same process except for the gun episode. Without this preparation, I could not have withstood the emotional onslaught of his dying.

Understanding and pride would have been even more evident in my father's eyes to learn that I'd found and accepted my own limitations and I'd *stopped* working with cancer patients, from time to time, when the burden was too heavy and burn-out too strong.

But bewilderment would have filled my father's eyes if he learned how I coped with those same limitations—by turning inward in prayer and outward to psychological counseling. He never did understand people talking about their problems, much less talking about them to strangers. That was the attitude of his era—"Pick yourself up and get *on* with it," he'd say. "Nobody can do it but you." Then he'd add, "By God, you don't have a corner on the market of misery."

He was wrong. Not about the "corner on the market of misery," but about doing it alone. The striving has to come from within, of course; yet I can't help but wonder how much pain would have been spared in his own life if he'd had a Fr. Tom or a Ken Kopel instead of Jack Daniels' to help him face his demons during those early years. And subsequently how much more pain would have been spared in my brother's life and in my own, and in the infinite extension of all those whose lives we touched. But through my father's eyes seeing a counselor would equate to yelling "calf-rope!"—or surrender. I almost surrendered—succumbed might be the better word— to the memory of that icy cold pistol jammed against my cheek, until Ken simply said, "Many strong men, when faced with their own painful struggles with death choose to take matters into their own hands, and try to take their own lives— you merely got in the way . . ."

I not only could accept that explanation, I could put the whole terrible, haunting episode behind me and *live*.

Undoubtedly, yelling "calf-rope" saved me. When I learned not to give up, but to give *in*—surrender to contemplation, to listening to what was inside me as Sr. Marie taught; surrender to "face the tiger" as Luthe taught, so its terrible roars and growls could not obscure the messages of contemplation; and then to surrender to surrendering, to say "Please help me," as my brother Patrick taught me—that's when I realized that I could not survive all by myself. Each of these messengers of survival were weavers of hope for me. If anyone of these treads of my own healing tapestry were missing, I don't quite know how I would have completed the pattern of survival.

But I know *why* I survived. Because I want, I *need* to tell you to stay the course—<u>*Endure*</u>. It *is* possible to do. Despite fear. Despite depression and family histories. Despite *all* odds.

There are those souls who will see, hear and understand your trial, those who will embrace but not carry you, who will encourage you and pull you forward out of your own cave of shadows and despair, and start you upon your own odyssey of light—*if* you are seeking them. *Ask . . . Seek . . . you will find.*

And you yourself will change from within. The immobilizing pain of depression and terror will surprise you one day and dissipate slowly, veil by veil, like a dark gray rolling fog in the morning sun. And out of that dawning stillness will come spiritual peace. And you will smile when you realize my father's words were absolutely straight-arrow when he said, *"The sun don't shine on the same dog's back ever' day—your turn's comin'."*

My turn has come. I've taken my first sunshine steps:

Paradoxically, I've stepped gingerly through the snow and ice of a dark, wondrously renewing New Year Celebration in Anchorage, Alaska, to begin this surprising, sunny time of my life. Ice and snow seem to form the chrysalis of my rebirth.

With some of these steps, I've descended a level of the Louvre Museum in Paris, mesmerized by the beauty and power of the Greek Nike, Victory of Samothrace—Winged Victory. That massive, ethereal sculpture has fascinated me since I studied it in Humanities twenty years earlier. I stood at the base of this amazing marble Nike and I could almost feel and hear the power of the wind against her wings. I felt the exultation of her victory and mine and I wept.

With other steps, I've forced myself to overcome my claustrophobia to climb cramped, narrow passageways of an ancient Irish castle in County Cork to suspend myself backwards, upside-down, to kiss the Blarney Stone. I'll have to warn my old friend Joe.

The same sunny steps have echoed as they carried me into the luminous, overpowering Cathedral at Chartres, past all the Biblical stories and saints sculpted around its altar and nave, bathed in the luminous, healing light of its rose windows, and then back, providentially, to an All Saints' Day Mass at Notre Dame Cathedral in Paris—a most solemn, high mass, with all its choirs singing from the upper levels blending soaring angelic voices with the ethereal thunder of the pipe organ. So majestic, so moving was this celebration, I felt I must have transcended and passed through Heaven's Portals. Once again as in Montreal's Notre Dame, awe filled my soul, but this time mixed with unspeakable gratitude because I no longer felt isolated, distanced from God. At long last, I understood. This desert daughter no longer wondered who and where the Great Spirit was.

This luminous new path has led me to the quiet shores of Maui, to Japanese friends who became as family to me—Maui, where I experienced another bigger, more mysterious family, two pods of humpback whales in Kapalua Bay, with a newborn calf being nurtured in the shallows by the mother and surrogate mother and felt privileged to witness such maternal tenderness. This shining path has led me back to explore what Salvatore calls the only mystical land left in this country—New Mexico—Santa Fe, Taos and the Sangre de Christo Mountains.

I've walked in solemn reverence through the soaring halls of the Palacio Nacional in Mexico City, stirred once again by the powerful murals of Diego Rivera that cry out for justice, and I've traveled for the first time down the humble streets of Malinalco, inland from Vera Cruz, meeting the warmth and generosity and beauty of this modest village's people and felt at one with each of them.

I have yet to journey to Macchupicchu, but do not regret it, for I am alive because of its land's finest gift.

Throughout these sunny days, this gift of years, I've seen many wonders, I've met unforgettable people, some of the world's great characters. But one extraordinary experience out-shines them all—I attended the celebration and birth of my Clinton, my son's son. Clinton Coore Johnson is the miracle I thought I'd never see, and somewhere my mother and my father are beaming at his boisterous arrival. He calls me "Lambie." One day he'll change this to "Grammie," I know, but for now "Lambie" is the sweetest sound I've ever heard.

Paradoxically, now instead of fear I'd die too young, I'm coping with growing older. With each successive phase of this process, I'm reminded of two key thoughts: The first from my Ft. Apache cowboy father, "Old age is not for sissies," and the second from Monsignor Tomas Cahalane of County Cork, Ireland, and Tucson, "As the body fails, the spirit grows."

I know they are true, for more than anything else, the odyssey of this desert daughter has taught me that I am more than flesh and blood and sinew, more even than fear and chemicals and body parts that betray.

Through my Father's Eyes, I am spirit and compassion and understanding and the joy of overcoming and Victory. I am a gleaning of Hope and Love. In my Father's Words, He makes *all things new.*

I am brand new.

Courage is knowing you will be.

Annotated Bibliography

Benson, H. *The Relaxation Response.* New York: William Morrow Co., 1975.

Brinker, Nancy and Harris, Catherine McEvily. *The Race is Run One Step at a Time.* New York: Simon & Schuster, 1990. *Includes comprehensive resource lists on breast cancer health care and information.*

Cameron, Judia and Bryan, Mark. *The Artist's Way: A Spiritual Path to Higher Creativity.* New York: Jeremy Tarcher/G.P. Putnam's Sons, 1992.
While not a book about cancer, this offers imaginative techniques for recovery.

Colgrove, Melba, Bloomfield, Harold H. and McWilliams, Peter. *How to Survive the Loss of a Love.* Los Angeles: Prelude Press, 1976.
Substitute the word "health" for "love" and this creative healing book offers a great guide for healing.

Cousins, Norman. *Anatomy of an Illness as Perceived by the Patient: Reflections on Healing and Regeneration.* New York: W.W. Norton, 1979.

———. *Head First: The Biology of Hope.* New York: E.P. Dutton, 1989.

Hutschnecker, A.A. T*he Will to Live*. New York: Thomas Y. Crowell Co., 1953.

Luthe, Wolfgang. *Creativity Mobilization Technique*. New York: Grune & Stratton, 1976.
This detailed textbook of the CMT process is best approached with an instructor.

Moyers, Bill. *Healing and the Mind*. New York: Doubleday & Co., 1993.

Simonton, O. Carl, Mathews-Simonton, Stephanie and Creighton, James L. *Getting Well Again*. Los Angeles: Jeremy Tarcher, 1978. *Still the single best book for survival, this provides excellent lifesaving techniques and guidance.*

Simonton, O. Carl, Henson, Reid and Hampton, Brenda. *The Healing Journey: The Simonton Center Program for Achieving Physical, Mental and Spiritual Health*. New York: Bantam Books, 1992.

William, Marriane. *Illuminata*. New York: Random House, Inc., 1994. *This author's prayers for healing, for guidance, for love and forgiveness provide a daily renewal for those of any faith on a spiritual quest.*

Appendix

Sharon Wanslee's 38 "Survival Rules"

Although all 38 Survival Rules are cited throughout the text, at the end of each chapter, it may be helpful to present them all again here, as an extended prayer of hope.

Survival Rule #1:

Now is the time to become more open, more receptive, more inquiring into the ways of hope and survival than you have ever before been in your life—you are entering a new and different world.

Survival Rule #2:

In the beginning you will experience shock and denial. A feeling of numbness will set in. This is okay. It's normal. Slow down and savor small moments as you go, and remember words from a wise, old cowpuncher—"Take 'er slow."

Survival Rule #3:

Listen to your own inner body knowledge. If I had waited to have my first mammogram until I was fifty, as the American Medical Association now recommends, I would *never* have had one. *I would already have been dead for fifteen years.*

Survival Rule #4:

A medical diagnosis of cancer can make you crazy. It's important to know that *this madness is normal.* There are many ways to deal with the craziness so that you can deal with the cancer—and win.

Survival Rule #5:

Build your own support group right away—family members, friends, therapists, clergy, co-workers, male and female—for it will be their love and their care that will give you strength for the battles, so that you may win your war. How do you do this? Simply ask them.

Survival Rule #6:

To guide you through this new, unchartered territory, buy two paperback books immediately—*Getting Well Again*, by O. Carl Simonton, M.D., and Stephanie Matthews-Simonton, the best step-by-step course through the challenge of cancer back to health, and *How to Survive the Loss of a Love*, by Colgrove, Bloomfield and McWilliams, a survival guide for the loss of anything—especially health.

Survival Rule #7:

Say a resounding "YES" to Life. Now more than ever be open to *new* ideas, methods of healing and wholeness. Explore *new* avenues to reach your goal—complete and vibrant wellness.

Survival Rule #8:

Anger, even rage, is a vital part of the recovery process. Allow the anger to rise, to spew out, so that it does not stay seething within, blocking the healing process. Your system needs all the equilibrium and strength it can find to heal you.

Deal with rage in productive ways. In the CMT process, one learns that the combination of large muscle movements and verbalizing is most conducive in neutralizing stress; i.e., long, stomping, curse-darn-swearing walks, throwing cheap dishes at a rock wall while voicing your anger.

Therapy—many kinds of therapy are good—art, dance, music therapy—and sometimes it's helpful to simply be alone and write out your pain and frustration about being betrayed by your own body. The CMT process proved most successful for me; up to that point it was the only acceptable place to vent my anger.

Whatever you do, DON'T SUFFER IN ANGELIC SILENCE. MARTYRS DO NOT SURVIVE.

Survival Rule #9:

Forgive yourself for "getting" cancer. Betrayal by one's own body is perhaps the ultimate—yet inevitable—treachery, but many factors entered into this medial equation. So be gentle with yourself. Nurture yourself and that spiritual side of you that will guide you to triumph.

Survival Rule #10:

Now is the time to eliminate as much "other stress" from your life as possible. Cancer is stress enough. "Other stress" includes disturbing situations, environments—even people. If annoying persons cannot be avoided, at least try to limit the amount of time spent with them. And if even this damage control is impossible, then greatly reward yourself later for your saintly patience in dealing with their particular poison.

One of the rewards might be to write about them in your journal and describe them in minute and exacting detailed caricature.

Survival Rule #11:

Get outside yourself. The fastest way to stop thinking about your fear, your pain, your misery is to talk to someone who is going through the same throes—or worse. Listen to them, help them in some way and do it often. Join a support group or simply look around the doctor's waiting room and *really see* the people there. Start a conversation. Life will surprise you with its comforting.

Survival Rule #12:

When the desire to live burns with such intensity that your every thought, every word, your very breath and heartbeat become a prayer to God and the Universe for healing, then and only then will your meditations, visualizations and dreams become truly at One with all your medical procedures and you will know Wholeness.

Survival Rule #13:

When you can turn and thank God for the graces coming into your life, not only *in spite of* what you are going through, but *because* of it, this is a great and healing "Yes! Yes! Yes!" response to Life.

Survival Rule #14:

Remember Luthe's words—
"You must face the tiger."

Survival Rule #15:

Love is the Great and Unequaled Comforter. If you have no one who loves you with unconditional acceptance, fine someone. They are there waiting for you—in your family, among your friends or acquaintances, in a support or prayer group. If, on assessment you realize you have no one, *get help fast*. Seek a counselor, priest, minister or psychologist and build from there.

If you still find no one who loves you, maybe you are not being lovable enough. Maybe you need to seek the second greatest comforter first—forgiveness. Forgive others. If you cannot find it in your heart to do it for them, do it for yourself. Without it there can be no true healing from within. Then forgive yourself. Forgiveness leads inevitably to Love.

Maybe you need the great unconditional lover—a dog—the best of all earthly examples of how to love and be loved.

Survival Rule #16:

Laughter is medicine. Aside from the endorphins it produces, laughter offers a surcease from the grip of pain, anxiety and fear. Indulge yourself with great doses of this wondrous elixir. If you are skeptical about laughter as painkiller and healer, read Norman Cousin's *Anatomy of an Illness* and *Head First: The Biology of Hope*. Test laughter for yourself.

Survival Rule #17:

The antidote to fear is not courage, but Love. Replace fear with Love. Courage will naturally follow.

Survival Rule #18:

Utmost confidence in your doctor is imperative. With it you can win. Without it, all the medical procedures in the world will be sabotaged by the lurking doubts in your mind. If you do not have such full trust, search until you find the physician not only worthy to be in charge of your prognosis, but of your hope as well.

Survival Rule #19:

Whine carefully. If you catalogue your woes aloud, there may be one listening who has been through much more. Or say to yourself, "That's just what they're saying in Bosnia"—or Rwanda or wherever the pocket of the world's misery happens to be at the time. This thought provides great leveling perspective to your own sufferings.

Save up real complaints to discuss with a counselor or a confidant. And choose these carefully.

Survival Rule #20:

Progress will be indicated by a zigzag line not a straight one. A few days of confidence and vitality may be followed by days of depression and total prostration. That's okay. It's all part of the healing process.

Never, NEVER assess your life, your situation, your medical prognosis at night. If you are already experiencing the dark night of your soul, don't plunge yourself deeper into the shadows. Too many fears are born in th gloom of exhaustion and discouragement.

Fill your evening and night hours with as much comfort, joy, love, laughter, rest and renewal as possible. Your body needs this time for healing purposes. Your mind and your soul need to be replenished by courage, goodness and peace.

Reserve time early in the morning every day to worry. Set an alarm for a half-hour. Write down each and every worry or dire thought you can imagine. When the alarm rings, slam the notebook shut. Put it and your fears away for another twenty-four hours. When your cancer challenge is over, you will be amazed at how few of those anxieties materialized.

Survival Rule #21:

Find a counselor worthy to be called True Friend. And if you can, see your counselor before any major treatment or medical procedure. This fortification will surprise you with its strength.

Then find a new notebook and reserve it for all those thoughts that are life-giving and filled with hope, for all those ideas that come to you while reaching out to Life, for funny sayings, cartoons or happenings, or for inspiring ones. Refer to it often. Call it your "Survival Journal."

Survival Rule #22:

"Stop postponing living."

Live fully in The Now. *This moment is all there is.* Live it wholly, heart, mind and soul.

Survival Rule #23:

The ultimate healing is death. Make peace with this reality and with the thought that none of us gets "outta this alive." But remember, as the body dies, the spirit grows. And so does Love. Love transcends Death.

Survival Rule #24:

Setbacks, even devastating ones, are inevitable in the painfully slow progress toward Victory. Don't anticipate them, but don't be thrown by them either. There will be a solution. Help will be found. Keep your eyes not on the setback, only on the prize of Victory.

Survival Rule #25:

Run away—for a little while. If pressures grow too great, if too much advice and too many decisions overwhelm you, and you are too depleted physically and emotionally to make sense of any of it, maybe you need to run away and find your own Corpus Christi.

Simply escape. Find time for peace and solitude. Then simply return prepared for another round of the cycle of healing.

Survival Rule #26:

No one—not one person—is meant to go through a cancer experience alone. Seek wisdom. Seek comfort. Seek peace. As a child of the Universe you have not only the right, but the responsibility to search for nurturing. Truly seek answers and truly listen when they come, whether from the clergy, loved ones, counselors or even chance remarks from strangers. You will know when words are meant for you and your healing.

Survival Rule #27:

Some mountains were never created to be scaled alone. When my brother and I were growing up our dad taught us many games which only ended when one of us yelled, "Calf rope!" meaning "I surrender."

As an adult fighting catastrophic disease, there comes a time when it is self-defeating to say in our childish manner, "I can do it all by myself." At these times the most healing words one can utter are "Calf rope!"

We know that Christ in his agony surrendered his will to God by saying, "Father, into your hands I commend my spirit." At some point in our lives we must be compelled to make the same life-changing decision—admit our absolute dependency on God and on our loved ones, father, mother, sister, brother or friend. Realize that it may be a gift to them to simply tell them, "I need you. Please help me."

Don't worry about repaying their kindness. The ultimate way to repay them is to help someone in need further on down the road.

Survival Rule #28:

There is no true healing of the body unless the mind and the soul also become whole. And it is exceedingly difficult to find peace, health and wholeness of the spirit amid the din of our daily existence.

Seek peace. Seek solitude in a quiet corner—an empty church is ideal—if only for a few moments each day. In the silence answers will come.

Survival Rule #29:

Whatever your religion or non-religion, when you take the time to get in touch with the spiritual side of your nature, with all that is most sacred in your life, the healing in your soul cannot help but be reflected in your physical health.

Survival Rule #30:

Seek until you find your own "Listening Heart."

Survival Rule #31:

Nature's beauty and rhythms can bring us back into harmony of soul, with each other and with all living things. Find a place apart where you can experience Nature, wildlife and that part of your own Life that is *not* tamed, civilized and packaged appropriately for polite society.

Break away. Travel to "see a different tree." What you will learn about your Oneness with the Universe will be vital to your healing.

Your place apart doesn't have to be "spiritual," but it is crucial for it to be a definite "retreat" from all that is usual, normal and routine. The spiritual aspect will follow.

Survival Rule #32:

Many years have passed since I found my "New Leaf." The more I have shared this story with others, the more I am convinced that this leaf is not really mine. Its message is for all of us—for you, in particular, who are reading these words at this very moment—"Behold, I make *all* things new" is the enduring promise. Grasp it. Believe it. Live it.

Survival Rule #33:

Everything you have learned as the patient of a catastrophic illness can be utilized as a caregiver.

No one ever faces the death of a loved one without also confronting feelings about their own mortality. Accept this. Consult Chapter 19 of *Getting Well Again*, "The Family Support System," and work with patience and love in your nurturing of others.

Survival Rule #34:

A patient needs to feel free to express any and all fears and emotions—both positive and negative—without fear of censure. Remember your own moments, days, of feeling alone and isolated, and do for the patient what you so desperately needed someone to do for you—listen quietly, understand and offer comfort and strength.

Survival Rule #35:

As Kathleen taught me, the single most important thing you can do for a patient is the simple act of being there. Just *be there* in their hour of sorrow and greatest need.

Survival Rule #36:

Understand that morphine and other pain-killing medications can alter a person's mind and emotions, their entire persona. And it is not at all unusual for men of great strength of mind and will to try to take their own life upon suffering their own terminal illness. Feeling totally out of control of their life, they "take control" of their own death.

Survival Rule #37:

Tombs *cannot* end Life or Love.

Survival Rule #38:

For the Abuser:
Get help. There are those who will understand your cry for help, who will accept you and set you free from the pain you carry that causes the pain you inflict.

For the Abused:
Find help for yourself. Find a method, some process or therapy that will lead you through understanding the pain of the abuser to ultimate forgiveness. Only then will you be healed.

And never, ever pass your pain to others. The pain must stop with you. And you must grow through it.

A Desert Daughter's Odyssey

ABOUT THE AUTHOR . . .

Sharon Wanslee is a native of Tucson. She grew up using as much Spanish as English. She graduated from the University of Arizona with the very highest honors, including the academic honorary society Phi Beta Kappa. She learned to speak and write elegant and lyrical French as well as Spanish and became an accomplished writer for newspapers and magazines. This is her first book.

www.ingramcontent.com/pod-product-compliance
Lightning Source LLC
Chambersburg PA
CBHW031502270326
41930CB00006B/216